ADOLESCENT HEALTH

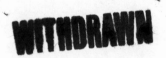

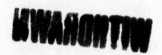

Adolescent Health

Policy, Science, and Human Rights

EDITED BY WILLIAM BOYCE,
JENNIFER ROCHE, AND DIANE DAVIES

Published for The Social Program Evaluation Group
Queen's University
by
McGill-Queen's University Press
Montreal & Kingston · London · Ithaca

© McGill-Queen's University Press 2009
ISBN-978-0-7735-3511-4 (cloth)
ISBN-978-0-7735-3525-1 (paper)

Legal deposit second quarter 2009
Bibliothèque nationale du Québec

Printed in Canada on acid-free paper that is 100% ancient forest free
(100% post-consumer recycled), processed chlorine free.

McGill-Queen's University Press acknowledges the support of the Canada
Council for the Arts for our publishing program. We also acknowledge
the financial support of the Government of Canada through the Book
Publishing Industry Development Program (BPIDP) for our publishing
activities.

Library and Archives Canada Cataloguing in Publication

Adolescent health: policy, science, and human rights / edited by
William Boyce, Jennifer Roche and Diane Davies.

Includes bibliographical references.
ISBN 978-0-7735-3511-4 (bnd)
ISBN 978-0-7735-3525-1 (pbk)

1. Teenagers – Health and hygiene – Canada. 2. Youth – Health and
hygiene – Canada. 3. Teenagers – Health and hygiene – Government
policy – Canada. 4. Youth – Health and hygiene – Government policy –
Canada. 5. Teenagers – Health and hygiene – Research – Canada.
6. Youth – Health and hygiene – Research – Canada. I. Boyce, William F.
(William Francis), 1949– II. Roche, Jennifer, 1968– III. Davies, Diane,
1969– IV. Queen's University (Kingston, Ont.). Social Program
Evaluation Group

RJ103.C3A36 2009   362.10835'0971   C2008-906619-7

Typeset in Sabon 10.5/13
by Infoscan Collette, Quebec City

Dedicated to Professor Alan J.C. King,
Faculty of Education, Queen's University

Contents

Tables and Figures

FIGURES

Preface

WILLIAM BOYCE

Concrete policy analysis and program development in adolescent health and well-being has lagged behind conceptual advances in adolescent neuro-behavioural issues and models of psychological development. This lag has been caused, in part, by a neglect of adolescence as a substantive focus for policy-making, unlike the focus on early childhood well-being, women's health, and (increasingly) men's health. There are also broader reasons for this gap, such as: insufficient resource allocations for health promotion in contrast to curative approaches; disagreements within the scientific community regarding the evidence base for adolescent health; tensions regarding the appropriate role for global ethical standards in local policy; the role of local communities in deciding policy priorities; and diverse interests within the policy process itself. This book addresses these broad concerns and focuses on often-expressed interests in comprehensive, coordinated policy for adolescence.

Spurred on by some recent advances in the early childhood field that have demonstrated the potential usefulness of an integrated approach to research and policy, there is keen interest in exploring a similar coordinated approach in adolescence. The general need for such an approach is clear, due to the transitional nature of adolescence between childhood and adulthood, the individual variability of developmental progress in adolescence, and the mixed responsibilities of multiple sectors and jurisdictions for adolescent health and well-being. Such an approach would theoretically allow the development of synergistic, non-contradictory, and mutually supportive policies and programs across sectors that could advance the health and well-being of Canadian youth. Whether such an integrated approach is possible or not, there is a real need for an analysis of the determinants of adolescent health and a comprehensive examination of the possibilities for coordinated policy and practices that are required to promote and protect adolescent health and prevent future problems in adulthood. The potential at this time in Canada for contributing to such an analysis, which could inform both adolescent health research priorities and policy development, has motivated this book.

Acknowledgments

We would like to acknowledge the unique and valuable role of Diane Davies in the early coordination of this book. We also are grateful for the generous financial contributions made by the Public Health Agency of Canada (through Mary Johnston) and by the Canadian Population Health Initiative of the Canadian Institute for Health Information.

PART ONE

Introduction

1

Background to Health Policy-making

WILLIAM BOYCE

ORIGINS OF THE HEALTH PROMOTION AND
POPULATION HEALTH MOVEMENTS IN CANADA

Since the 1970s, the Government of Canada has been searching for
a new direction in health beyond the provision of health care and
in line with the World Health Organization's definition of health as
"a state of complete physical, mental, and social well-being, and not
merely the absence of disease or infirmity" (WHO 1946, 1). The
WHO's 1986 Ottawa Charter, the result of the First International
Conference on Health Promotion, which was held in Canada's capital, led the way in conceptualizing health promotion as an essential
adjunct to health services, health protection, and prevention strategies. The Charter defined health promotion as "the process of
enabling people to increase control over, and to improve, their
health" (WHO 1986, 1), although it was unclear whether such participation was intended to be a means to health or an end in itself.
The social determinants of health, such as social support, education,
and income, were also in vogue at this time, so that health promotion was envisioned as a multifaceted strategy, including: (a) strengthening community action, (b) developing personal skills, (c) reorienting
health services, (d) building healthy public policy, (e) creating supportive environments, and (f) enabling, mediating, and advocating.
The broader goals of health promotion were to improve social environments, integrate the social determinants of health with public
policy, and facilitate community participation. Although Canada's
performance in these areas has been modest (e.g., Pederson et al.
1988 regarding public policy and Boyce 2001 regarding community

Table 1.1
Canada's determinants of health, 1994 and 2003

1994[1]	2003[2]
• Income and social status • Social support networks • Education • Employment and working conditions • Safe and clean physical environments • Biology and genetic make-up • Personal health practices and coping skills • Childhood development • Health services	• Income and social status • Social support networks • Education and literacy • Employment/working conditions • Social environments • Physical environments • Personal health practices and coping skills • Healthy child development • Biology and genetic endowment • Health services • Gender • Culture

Sources:
[1] Federal, Provincial, and Territorial Advisory Committee on Population Health. 1994. *Strategies for Population Health: Investing in the Health of Canadians.* Report prepared for the Meeting of the Ministers of Health, Halifax, Nova Scotia, 14–15 September 1994. Ottawa, Ontario: Health Canada. http://www.phac-aspc.gc.ca/ph-sp/phdd/pdf/e_strateg.pdf. Retrieved 5 December 2006.
[2] Public Health Agency of Canada. 2003. *Santé de la population/Population Health: What determines health?* http://www.phac-aspc.gc.ca/ph-sp/phdd/determinants/index.html#determinants. Retrieved 17 November 2006.

participation of disadvantaged persons), it has shown an eagerness to experiment with new concepts – and to a lesser extent structures – that could facilitate health. The Canadian federal health bureaucracy has led the way in these health promotion efforts (Boyce 2002), fundamentally changing the role of health professionals in the new approach (Pederson et al. 1988).

While these strategies for health promotion were being defined and tested, Canada's health goals were also being refined to address an expanded set of health determinants. In the 1990s, Canada and other countries began to support a broader population health concept, which pointed to determinants of health as key causes of health inequalities across entire populations (Evans, Barer, and Marmor 1994). This perspective recognized the effect of factors other than genetics, health services, and behavioural choices on health status, in particular the influence of social, economic, political, and physical environments. In 1994, Health Canada articulated the interrelated determinants of health (see Table 1.1).

The population health movement facilitated a conceptual leap from disease prevention (emphasizing individual risk reduction) and health promotion (encouraging social policy and participation) to advancement of population health (emphasizing determinants or structural settings and conditions that contributed to general health and well-being) (Ziglio, Levin, and Bertinato 1998). The population inequalities approach focused attention on those groups most at risk of poor health and added gender and culture to Health Canada's list of health determinants (see Table 1.1; also, Bhatti and Hamilton 2002). Although increased recognition of the social determinants of health played a key role in both the evolution of health promotion and the genesis of the population health movement, health promotion (which is characterized by grassroots community action and participatory and qualitative research) has viewed public policy as only one of six strategies for action (enumerated above), while population health (which is characterized by research and policy partnerships based on scientific evidence and large-scale datasets) has often given preference to public policy over other strategies (Lavis 2002). This book examines the fruits of this population health approach (also known as the population inequalities approach) and its role in health policy development with respect to adolescents. Let us now consider some definitions and typologies of health policy.

WHAT IS HEALTH POLICY?

Health policy, in the broadest sense, is understood as the actions of government and other players aimed at maintaining and improving a population's state of health. Distinctions can also be made between health care policy, prevention policy, and intersectoral (or integrated) policy (Spasoff 1999). Health policy includes courses of action that affect the set of institutions, organizations, services, and funding arrangements of the health care system. In many views, however, policy goes beyond health services to include actions by public, private, and voluntary organizations that have an impact on health (Walt 1994, 41).

Two contrasting, and nuanced, interpretations of health policy are:

(a) An authoritative statement of intent adopted by governments on behalf of the public with the aim of improving the health and welfare of the population; that is, a centrally determined basis for action.

(b) What health agencies actually do rather than what governments would like them to do (Palfrey 2000). In Palfrey's interpretation, health policy is determined by observation of the outcomes of decision making rather than by government intention.

Theorist Ted Lowi (1964) distinguishes between three traditional types of government policy. *Distributive* policies provide specific benefits to groups without regard to limited resources (e.g., Canada provides universal access to insured health services). *Regulatory* policies provide benefits to only some groups on the basis of a general rule (e.g., in Ontario, the purchase of alcohol is restricted to those aged nineteen years and older). *Redistributive* policies provide benefits to some by extending losses, often through taxation, to others (e.g., prescription drug coverage in Ontario is provided for seniors and those on welfare). Regulatory and redistributive policies are based on a recognition that there are persistent inequalities between populations either in terms of individuals' capacities (which need to be managed) or in terms of available resources (which need to be supplemented).

The definition that we ultimately assert in this book holds that not only is policy "an authoritative statement of intent by governments" but also one that should be reflective of the involvement of many stakeholders and that acknowledges the importance of closing the gap between intent and outcome. Governments arrive at policies through application of different models of policy-making, some of which we will now outline.

THE POLICY PROCESS

Charles Lindblom (1959) famously described the process of policy-making as "muddling through." A more optimistic view, expressed by Pederson et al. (1988) in writing about public health policy, is that policy formulation is a process of problem solving characterized by negotiation, bargaining, and collaboration among various actors with different interests, influence, and power.

According to Hall (1996), health inequalities between populations allow for three general influences on the policy-making process: ideas, interests, and institutions. The first influence on policy, *ideas*, includes research, evidence, other types of information, and the core principles of policy-makers, stakeholders, and the public. The second influence, *interests*, includes perceptions of who will benefit from, and who will be hurt by, any given policy. The third influence, *institutions*, includes factors such as policy history and various government decision-making characteristics such as transparency of the process, time pressures to take action, and the level of approval (legislative or executive) required to formalize policy. Research, and other evidence, is used principally to establish ideas for policy. Obviously, and as reflected in this book, policy does not depend on research alone but relies as well on contested principles, negotiated resources, and public pressure.

William Coleman (1985) employs a similar typology to characterize the process of policy-making in Canada: the problem stream, the politics stream, and the policy stream. The *problem stream* – that is, that which presents itself as an issue to be addressed – refers to the way in which government officials learn about social conditions requiring legislative action. The problem stream may involve the use of research evidence and statistical indicators, feedback from existing programs, or focusing events that may include some kind of crisis (e.g., the 1999 school shooting incident in Taber, Alberta). The *politics stream* represents: (a) the visible policy participants, the organized interests who highlight a problem and use the media to get attention and who can be inside or outside government; and (b) the hidden participants (consultants, researchers, or academics) who can leak information to the press or call attention to problems through scientific articles. The *policy stream* characterizes the methods of policy-makers who then select from among various problems and issues for action, using criteria such as congruence with existing values; anticipation of future constraints; public acceptability; politicians' receptivity; and technical feasibility in implementation.

Coleman predicts that policy is more likely to be formulated and implemented in Canada given the following conditions:

- the policy will not generate strong reaction, or the government can dissipate reaction;
- the change is marginal (or incremental) rather than fundamental;
- the goals of the policy are clearly stated, featuring one major objective;
- the policy is perceived to be based on a clear theory of cause and effect (i.e., perceived as a "good" policy and likely to succeed);
- the policy has relatively simple technical features (i.e., necessary knowledge and technology already exist);

Table 1.2
Pless's four-stage typology of policy development (1995)

The four stages of policy development are as follows:
1 Defining the magnitude, complexity, or social significance of a problem (through research)
2 Analyzing whether the issue is within the legislative authority of the policy body (through information)
3 Determining whether feasible solutions exist (through research)
4 Analyzing whether, on balance, the policy should be adopted, often using an interest group assessment (through information)

Source: Pless, I.B. 1995. *Crossing the Bridge: From Research to Child Health Policy*. Montreal: McGill University.

- adequate time and resources are seen to be available;
- the policy can be implemented by one actor or a few actors and does not depend on extensive networks of collaboration or coordination; and
- the policy can be introduced quickly and is therefore less likely to encounter opposition, resistance, or leadership changes.

Coleman suggests that if the problem, politics, and policy streams all come together, then policy action is more likely. That is, policy is more likely to get on the agenda if a government thinks that the issue is highly legitimate and feasible to implement and if the government has the support and trust of the public.

One last example of a policy-making typology that we wish to present is that of Dr Barry Pless, the well-known injury researcher, who, in a book on the development of child health policy in Canada (1995), describes four stages of policy development in which research evidence and information are required (these stages are listed in Table 1.2). This typology comprises the field of policy analysis, and a discussion of its shortcomings and possibilities for improvement (with regard to increasing use of scientific evidence on the part of policy-makers) is featured in Chapter 11 of this book.

·TWO FRAMEWORKS FOR POLICY-MAKING

Policy, then, and the policy-making process are extremely complex in nature. Let us now turn to the international context. The policy community worldwide is faced with both increased requirements for broad consultation with stakeholders and conditions of rapid change, creating a situation that is marked by insufficient time for effective policy development. Policy and program developers find themselves in need of new ideas and frameworks, increased resources, and clear guidelines.

Scientific approaches have been promoted by the health research establishment as providing ideas and rational evidence that may help to guide policy. At the same time, however, the multiple forces comprising globalization – not only those with respect to economies but also those concerning culture, security, and moral values as represented in various United Nations agreements – have assumed greater importance for policy-makers in every jurisdiction. Both of these influences – scientific evidence and abstract principles – are reflected in the policy-making typologies described by Hall (1996) and Coleman (1985). It could be argued that Pless's typology (1995), although overtly focused on the role of evidence in policy development, allows for the influence of principles and values in Stage 1 (social significance) and Stage 4 (interest group assessment).

Evidence-based policy-making and principled policy-making are two dominant frameworks that have been promoted to guide the development of adolescent health policy. This book presents an examination of how these two frameworks have been or may be applied, their respective shortcomings, the ways in which they may be combined for the creation of more comprehensive and complete policies, and the areas in which they potentially conflict.

OVERVIEW OF CONTENT

In Part I, we outline the need for evidence-based adolescent health policy. In addition to our description of the policy development process, we also indicate how a global agreement on human rights principles – the United Nations Convention on the Rights of the Child – is intended to be used to assist in the process of principled policy-making. In Part II, each of the chapters, all of which have been written by leaders in their fields, addresses a key issue in adolescent health and well-being, using Canadian adolescent health data (including data from the WHO Health Behaviour in School-Aged Children survey) to outline settings, conditions, and behaviours that affect adolescent health outcomes. Current key policy initiatives concerning adolescent health determinants or behaviours are reviewed in an effort to identify unresolved policy problems and to illuminate instances in which programs and policies have effectively used research analyses and a principled approach. Each chapter makes recommendations for future policy development in adolescent health, based on the coordination of scientific research and offering examples of successful policies in the field. The concluding chapters examine the following: the possibilities for a coordinated adolescent health research agenda; the opportunities and risks in focusing global agreements, such as the Convention on the Rights of the Child, on development of local adolescent health policy; the translation and use of research evidence in adolescent health policy fields; and the challenges in developing a comprehensive vision of adolescent health policy.

INTENDED USE OF THIS BOOK

The goal of this book is to further the thinking of scientists, policy-makers, and program planners by providing a detailed discussion of the adolescent health policy-making process from the perspectives of two frameworks: a principled framework based on the United Nations Convention on the Rights of the Child and an evidence-based framework based on current available research, with attention paid to determinants of health.

The book is intended to increase the interest in, and advance the coordination of action by governments and others towards, improving the health of adolescents. It will be of particular use to academics in the fields of psychology, sociology, social work, public health, education, medicine, and nursing who could use the information as a basic data source and as a resource for the development of a conceptual framework that incorporates international rights obligations and the complex web of health determinants for further analysis and debate. It is useful as a text or resource for college and university courses in health psychology, health education, health policy, and the social sciences. It will also be useful in helping legal and policy analysts, policy developers, program planners, and evaluators who may be working at the national, provincial, territorial, and local health unit levels to assess current adolescent policies and programs. An international audience, particularly in Europe and the United States, but also in other developed areas (such as Australia and the Far East), may be interested in the book's application of research evidence and global frameworks to improve adolescent health policy initiatives.

REFERENCES

Bhatti, T., and N. Hamilton. 2002. Health promotion: What is it? *Health Policy Research Bulletin* 1(3):5–7.

Boyce, W.F. 2001. Disadvantaged persons' participation in health promotion projects: Some structural dimensions. *Social Science and Medicine* 52(10):1551–64.

– 2002. Influence of health promotion bureaucracy on community participation: A Canadian case study. *Health Promotion International* 17:61–8.

Coleman, W.D. 1985. *Business and Politics: A Study in Collective Action*. Montreal: McGill-Queen's University Press.

Evans, R.G., M.L. Barer, and T.R. Marmor, eds. 1994. *Why Are Some People Healthy and Others Not?* New York: Aldine De Gruyter.

Hall, P.A. 1996. *Politics and Markets in the Industrialized Nations: Interests, Institutions and Ideas in Comparative Political Economy*. Cambridge, MA: Harvard University, Center for European Studies.

Lavis, J.N. 2002. Ideas at the margin or marginalized ideas? Non-medical determinants of health in Canada. *Health Affairs* 21(2):107–12.

Lindblom, C.E. 1959. The science of "muddling through." *Public Administration Review* 19:79–88.

Lowi, T. 1964. American business, public policy, case studies, and political theory. *World Politics* 16:677–713.

Palfrey, C. 2000. *Key Concepts in Health Care Policy and Planning*. London: MacMillan Press.

Pederson, A., R. Edwards, M. Kelner, V.M. Marshall, and K.R. Allison. 1988. *Coordinating Healthy Public Policy: An Analytic Literature Review and Bibliography*. Ottawa: Minister of Supply and Services.

Spasoff, R. 1999. *Epidemiologic Methods for Health Policy*. New York: Oxford University Press.

Walt, G. 1994. *Health Policy: An Introduction to Process and Power*. London: Zed Press.

World Health Organization. 1946. *Constitution*. Adopted 22 July. http://www.who.int/about/en/. Retrieved 17 November 2006.

– 1986. *Ottawa Charter for Health Promotion*. Copenhagen: World
  Health Organization Regional Office for Europe. http://www.who.int/
  health promotion/conferences/previous/ottawa/en/index.html. Retrieved
  17 November 2006.
Ziglio, E., L. Levin, and L. Bertinato. 1998. Social and economic
  determinants of health: Implications for promoting the health of
  the public. *Forum Trends in Experimental and Clinical Medicine*
  8(3):6–16.

2

Principled Policy-making:
The United Nations Convention
on the Rights of the Child

EMILY BOYCE

The fifty-four articles of the United Nations Convention on the Rights of the Child (UNCRC) comprise an international treaty that codifies the human rights and freedoms of every child, defined as every person under the age of eighteen years (United Nations 1989). In its preamble, the Convention reaffirms the principles proclaimed in the UN's own Charter: that recognition of the inherent dignity and equal and inalienable rights of all members of the human family is the foundation of freedom, justice, and peace in the world; and that the family is the fundamental unit of society and the natural environment for the growth and well-being of children.

The Convention was accepted by the UN General Assembly in 1989 and signed by 160 countries, including Canada, at the World Summit for Children in 1990. The treaty was ratified by Canada in 1991 and has since been ratified by 191 of the 193 UN member states (with the notable exceptions of the United States and Somalia). The years that followed ratification saw an unprecedented global focus on children's rights.

EFFECT OF UN INSTRUMENTS ON STATE POLICY-MAKING AND MONITORING

Canada's focus on child rights as a framework for policy-making is linked to its ratification of the UN Convention . It is therefore necessary to understand the nature of UN conventions and other instruments.

Previous international declarations of the rights of children exist (i.e., at Geneva in 1924 and the United Nations in 1959), as do official UN documents containing rules or principles relevant to children; however, none of these has been legally binding. Documents known as "declarations" act as proposals for future conventions, and they contain recommendations and suggestions for human rights definitions and convention articles. "Rules," "codes of conduct," "guidelines," and "principles" are all intended to stimulate action on the part of governments. These represent minimum conditions and standards accepted by the United Nations but are not intended to describe a model system for human rights. The enforcement of rules or principles is the responsibility of nations, not the UN; and the observance of rules, codes of conduct, principles, or guidelines is only legally binding where these are incorporated into national legislation. Adherence to UN rules or principles is therefore the prerogative of individual states. There is no formal obligation to comply (Bazilli 2000).

By contrast, conventions – known interchangeably as covenants or treaties – create legally binding international obligations for signatory member states that define their mutual duties and obligations. When national governments ratify UN conventions, they commit to adopting laws, policies, and measures to implement the rights stated therein. Special UN committees are created, with the adoption of such treaties, to monitor and evaluate states' progress in implementing convention articles. Upon ratification, states agree to submit progress reports or objective evaluations of their progress in implementing the treaty (United Nations High Commissioner for Human Rights 2006).

For example, under Article 44 of the Convention on the Rights of the Child (United Nations 1989), signatories agree to submit regular reports to a body known as the UN Committee on the Rights of the Child. Initial implementation reports are to be submitted within two years of ratification of the Convention and thereafter every five years. The Committee reviews the states' reports in consultation with officials of the respective states' governments. The aim of these consultations is to define problems, discuss what corrective measures should be taken, and invoke public commitments and decisions by governments to improve the situation. At the end of the process, the Committee adopts "concluding observations" which are widely publicized. Publicity, open debate, and international responses to these concluding observations serve to encourage and/or pressure governments to implement Committee suggestions for improvement.

The UN Convention on the Rights of the Child is the first document of its kind to invoke both commitment and accountability regarding child rights among ratifying governments. The Convention was therefore a major victory for human rights activists, non-government organizations, and other child rights advocates.

KEY CONVENTION PRINCIPLES

The Convention is based on four general principles formulated in Articles 2, 3, 6, and 12 (United Nations 1989). Article 2 expresses the principle of "non-discrimination," or equality of opportunity for all children to enjoy their rights. Article 3 contains the principle of "best interests of the child," with respect to decisions made by courts of law, administrative authorities, legislative bodies, and public and private social welfare institutions. Article 6 addresses the "inherent right to life" and "to the maximum extent possible the survival and development of the child," referring to children's basic physical health and survival and implying broader concern for other forms of personal and social development. Article 12 describes the principle of "the views of the child," stating that those views should be given "due weight in accordance with the age and maturity of the child." According to the United Nations, these four principles should guide interpretation of the Convention as a whole and, in so doing, inform the development and implementation of programs and policies (United Nations High Commissioner for Human Rights 2006).

Following from these four principles, the Convention can be seen as containing three broad categories of rights: the right to survival and development, to protection, and to participation. These rights include: provision of adequate resources for survival and proper development, such as food, shelter, clean water, health care, and formal primary education; protection from all forms of harm, such as physical abuse, violence, and exploitation; and participation, without discrimination, in exercising rights, such as taking part in decision making and speaking up on matters that directly affect their lives and futures.

Clearly, these principles and broadly defined sets of rights are open to interpretation. This attribute can be advantageous because it gives governments sufficient latitude to develop appropriate policies. On the other hand, failure to interpret or contextualize these principles in a way that reflects the many needs of a diverse child population, which includes adolescents, can lead to inadequate or biased policy. The Convention has been called a "text without a context" by some analysts, who underscore the importance of considering the cultural and social-ecological contexts of children's lives in policy and programming (Cook 2003, 7; Williams 2005, 4). In Canada – where adolescents and younger children come from a diversity of socio-political jurisdictions, local community contexts, ethnic backgrounds, social and economic classes, and family types – this attention to local and cultural context is key to the development of relevant and effective rights-based policy. As we see below, there are also some inherent tensions between concepts found in the Convention, and these require critical consideration when developing policy based on its principles.

THE CONCEPT OF CHILDREN'S "EVOLVING CAPACITIES"

Article 1 of the Convention defines the child as "every human being below the age of eighteen years unless[,] under the law applicable to the child, majority is attained earlier" (United Nations 1989). The Convention emphasizes child protection, but it also makes reference to the relevance of age and maturity and the "evolving capacities of the child" in the exercise of rights. Article 5 recognizes the rights and duties of parents to provide appropriate direction and guidance to the child in the exercise of rights "in a manner consistent with the evolving capacities of the child." Article 12 refers to the child's right to express opinions and be heard in matters affecting his or her life, in accordance with "age and maturity." Article 14 provides for the child's right to freedom of thought, conscience, and religion and for the parents' right and duty to provide guidance in a manner consistent with the child's "evolving capacities." Overall, the "evolving capacities of the child" are to be taken into consideration when it is decided how, when, and to what extent a child can exercise his or her rights independent of parents or guardians.

The inclusion of the right to participation makes the Convention not only the most comprehensive statement of child rights but also the target of some critics who fear that it may undermine the authority of parents and schools or that it may legitimize undesirable youth activities, such as gang membership. This is an inaccurate and unfortunate interpretation. The Convention emphasizes responsibilities as well as rights and, throughout, clearly and repeatedly upholds the importance of parents' roles. It states that governments must respect the responsibility of parents for providing appropriate guidance to their children, including guidance as to how children shall exercise their rights.

PROBLEMS OF INTERPRETATION FOR ADOLESCENT HEALTH

Apart from Articles 5, 12, and 14, however, the Convention makes no other mention of children's "evolving capacities," nor does it make further reference to how rights might be thought about in terms of the unique developmental stage of adolescence. Other articles refer to children's rights regarding "participation," though without reference to adolescents in particular, and these include Articles 13 (freedom of expression), 15 (freedom of association), 17 (access to information and media), 23 (social integration and participation of children with disabilities), and 31 (cultural, leisure, artistic and recreational activity). Despite these articles, however, the Convention is dominated by the language of protection, with nuances characterizing the state and family as care providers. The Convention reads principally as a document outlining the need to protect young children from violations of their rights and the need for states and families to ensure the maximum survival and development of young children.

It takes a great deal of interpretation and imagination to properly apply the Convention to the social problems of adolescents (e.g., unemployment, poverty, street life, independent living, sexuality, reproductive health, substance abuse, high-risk behaviours, suicide, peer relations, peer violence, and gendered violence) and their rights (e.g., their right to social security and a decent standard of living and their rights as young parents or persons with a disability). Chapter 13 attempts to examine some of these issues.

It is not difficult to see, then, why policy initiatives and evaluations based on the framework provided by the Convention on the Rights of the Child have tended to focus on early childhood development and the protection of younger children rather than on adolescent rights and participation. In Canada, for example, the Convention has increasingly served as a reference for child policy development and evaluation. It supplies the framework for Brighter Futures:

Canada's Action Plan for Children (launched in 1992 as a response to the World Summit for Children in 1990), the National Children's Agenda (launched in January 1997), and for a range of new policy and program initiatives arising from these action plans (Department of Canadian Heritage 1994; 2001). More recently, the Convention has been used to inform a national plan of action called A Canada Fit for Children (launched in May 2004), which is the government's official response to commitments made at the United Nations General Assembly Special Session on Children in 2002 (Government of Canada 2004).

Canada has a formal responsibility to comply with the Convention, but the use of a macro-level framework to direct policy-making and to assess policy has limitations. The Convention sets out broad, basic standards for child rights but lacks clear definitions or standards with which to evaluate whether policy truly meets the diverse needs of both adolescents and younger children. This becomes particularly apparent when the Convention is used to frame or evaluate policy related to adolescent health and well-being.

The Convention contains potentially conflicting principles of equity, protection, development, and participation, despite these being considered indivisible. This tension is analyzed in detail in Chapter 13. It also lacks clear definitions with regard to what constitutes an "adolescent," and it is unclear with regard to how states are to allow for children's "evolving capacities" and their "participation" in the exercise of rights or decisions (as opposed to simply having their rights "protected" by the state). This problem has made policy-making at once complicated and limited in the area of adolescent health. Finally, the UN Convention on the Rights of the Child's emphasis on overall youth policy-making and assessment may have further entrenched the invisibility the specific needs and concerns of adolescents. The Convention, with its focus on young children, may be contributing to the neglect of adolescence as a substantive or productive target for policy-making or scientific research.

THE POTENTIAL ROLE OF
THE CONVENTION IN GUIDING CANADIAN
"BIG PICTURE" RESEARCH AND POLICY

In Canada, the Convention on the Rights of the Child's lack of specificity is compounded by a lack of evidence-based research on the determinants of adolescent health. Scientific findings are often incomplete and can be misleading because the determinants of adolescent health often have multiple and interacting effects on outcomes. For example, family support and peer support may have different effects for adolescent independence seeking, mental health, and school connectedness – all of which may be valued outcomes in various program and policy contexts. A comprehensive understanding of the complexity and interactions between a range of health outcomes and their relations to health determinants is needed to ensure effective policy development. Unfortunately, effective coordination of different research streams pertaining to adolescent health has not yet occurred.

While today the government aspires to evidence-based policy-making, this impetus must be carefully monitored to ensure that it does not deteriorate into policy-making based on "whatever works" according to incompletely articulated criteria. In such circumstances, the tendency could be to adopt initiatives from other countries (often the United States or the United Kingdom) and to try to apply them to Canada. The problem with this pragmatic "whatever works" approach to policy-making is that it produces plenty of initiatives but no single vision that uniquely fits the Canadian experience. Consequently, policy-makers have been increasingly attracted to the Convention on the Rights of the Child and similar treaties in order to guide "big picture" research.

Nonetheless, in most cases, principled policy that is based on human rights is a secondary, after-the-fact consideration. Furthermore, there may be problems with regard to relevance and application of rights approaches to specific populations and contexts. It is easy to make general policy links explicit or meaningful in Canada as these human rights principles are founded on a Western understanding of basic freedoms and responsibilities; but it may be more difficult to make these same principles applicable to specific adolescent health contexts in non-Western settings.

Chapter 13 examines the tensions between the rights to development, protection, and participation when applied to the context of adolescent health. It then selects four broad determinants of adolescent health – violence, substance use, social inequality, and health promotion – and provides a much-needed analysis of each. In so doing, it considers both rights and evidence with an aim to making recommendations for policy.

REFERENCES

Bazilli, Susan. 2000. A brief guide to international human rights law for Canadian advocates. *Canadian Woman Studies* 20(3):64–71.

Cook, P. 2003. Cross-cultural perspectives on the child image. Presentation at the International Interdisciplinary Course on Children's Rights, Ghent, Belgium, 11–18 December. http://web.uvic.ca/iicrd/graphics/Cross-Cultural%20Perspectives%20on%20the%20Child%20Image%20–Ghent%20Pres.%2011.12.2003.pdf. Retrieved 17 October 2006.

Department of Canadian Heritage. 1994. *Canada's First Report on the Convention on the Rights of the Child.* Submitted to the UN, 17 June. Ottawa: Human Rights Program, Department of Canadian Heritage, Government of Canada. http://www.pch.gc.ca/progs/pdp-hrp/docs/crc/index_e.cfm. Retrieved 17 October 2006.

– 2001. *Canada's Second Report on the Convention on the Rights of the Child.* Submitted to the UN, 26 April. Ottawa: Human Rights Program, Department of Canadian Heritage, Government of Canada. http://www.pch.gc.ca/progs/pdp-hrp/docs/crc/index_e.cfm. Retrieved 17 October 2006.

Government of Canada. 2004. A Canada fit for children. Press release by the Government of Canada, 10 May. http://www.canadiancrc.com/Canadian_governments_plan_2004.htm. Retrieved 17 October 2006.

United Nations. 1989. *Convention on the Rights of the Child.* Geneva: United Nations.

United Nations High Commissioner for Human Rights. 2006. *Fact Sheet No. 10 (Rev. 1): The Rights of the Child.* Geneva, Switzerland: Office of the United Nations High Commissioner for Human Rights. http://www.ohchr.org/english/about/publications/docs/fs10.htm. Retrieved 17 October 2006.

Williams, Suzanne. 2005. *Meeting Canada's Obligations under the UN Convention on the Rights of the Child: From Paper Concepts to Living Benefits for Children.* Brief to Canada's Senate Committee on Human Rights, 21 February. Victoria, British Columbia: International Institute for Child Rights and Development (IICRD), Centre for Global Studies, University of Victoria. http://web.uvic.ca/iicrd/graphics/IICRDBrieftoSenateCommittee(final).pdf. Retrieved 17 October 2006.

3

Evidence-based Policy-making: Adolescent Health Research

IRVING ROOTMAN AND WILLIAM BOYCE

FUNCTIONAL DEFINITION OF EVIDENCE

This book looks at the role of evidence in adolescent health policy-making, so it is important that we consider the meaning of evidence. The term is often contested. It is used differently by various people, and it is sometimes used in a way that is intended to discredit those who have an important role to play in the policy-making context. McQueen and Anderson (2001) discuss the issue of defining "evidence" in depth in a book that deals with evaluation in health promotion. Among the definitions of the term "evidence" are:

- "[Something a]pparent, manifest, obvious, palpable, clear, plain";
- "Something that has occurred with certainty";
- "The product of observation"; and
- "The product of experiment." (McQueen and Anderson 2001, 64–65).

These definitions range from the colloquial to the scientific. McQueen and Anderson note that literature in the history and philosophy of science does not contain extensive discussion of the term. For example, in the field of evidence-based medicine, the word "evidence" remains without specification and definition. They further discuss the relevance of the concept for health promotion and put forth a cogent argument as to why it may be an inappropriate idea in much of the health promotion field. McQueen and Anderson suggest that in science the rules of evidence are tied to specific disciplines.

Health promotion, though, is a multidisciplinary field, which makes it difficult to determine which rules of evidence should be used.

This debate is, however, to some extent moot as it is clear that the term will continue to be used in the field, as is indicated by the fact that the 1998 World Health Assembly passed a resolution calling for "evidence-based health promotion," including both quantitative and qualitative sources. In addition, other writers active in the field, such as Keith Tones, have endorsed the concept and argued in favour of a "judicial" approach, by which he means "providing evidence which would lead a jury to committing themselves to take action even when 100% proof is not available" (1997, 3).

A judicial approach may also be applicable in the health policy field, which leaves open the possibility of recognizing the value of a variety of types of evidence, ranging from the experimental to the experiential. The trick is to weight this evidence appropriately and to integrate it into the policy process in a rigorous and meaningful manner, along with other important considerations, such as resource availability, that must inevitably be taken into account. Thus, a definition of evidence that we propose, in the context of adolescent health policy development, is: systematically collected and rigorously analyzed information pertinent to the health of adolescents.

THREE CONTRIBUTIONS OF HEALTH RESEARCH TO POLICY

Health research has three objectives that can contribute to adolescent health policy development. These objectives are central to the scientific method, yet they also fall within Pless's four-stage typology of policy development (1995) as presented in Table 1.2 of this book. First, research can establish common patterns of population health status, or health outcomes, to help determine the need for interventions. Second, research can establish patterns of health determinants that contribute to these outcomes to explain the biological and social mechanisms that produce health. Third, research can establish the effectiveness of interventions to improve health status or prevent problematic outcomes.

The first objective of research, determination of adolescent health status, is being strengthened considerably in Canada through various cross-sectional and prevalence studies, such as the Health Behaviour in School-Aged Children (HBSC) study, the National Longitudinal

Table 3.1
Influence of various health determinants on early deaths (but not morbidity)
on a population basis: Example of a longitudinal study from the United States

Behavioural patterns	40%
Genetic predispositions	30%
Social circumstances	15%
Physical environment	5%
Shortfalls in medical care	10%

Source: McGinnis, J.M., P. Williams-Russo, and J.R. Knickman. 2002. The case for more active
policy attention to health promotion. Health Affairs 21(2):78–93.

Survey of Children and Youth (NLSCY), the National Population
Health Survey (NPHS), and the General Social Survey (GSS). The
advantage of repeated cycles of these studies is that researchers can
introduce new topical areas of investigation as required.

The second objective of research, identifying determinants and
causal mechanisms of adolescent health, is proceeding cautiously
and requires longitudinal studies (such as the NLSCY) that repeat
measures over time in the same individuals. Unfortunately, longitudinal studies cannot easily shift emphasis to address new emerging
social or environmental issues; nonetheless, these studies can reveal
the relative influence of various adolescent health determinants in
Canada, allowing intensive investigation of key areas.

Sample results of a longitudinal study from the United States are
presented in Table 3.1, which shows the influence of various health
determinants on early deaths. The health of any population is the
product of the intersecting influences of these domains, which vary
in their impact depending on when they occur in the life cycle and
upon the particular constellation of preceding and succeeding factors.
This type of information gives some idea of policy priority in the
United States, with behavioural patterns (and their particular determinants and moderators) being of high importance for mortality.
Obviously, the influence of these domains on adolescent mortality/
morbidity in Canada would be different. Attention to the determinants
of non-mortality outcomes is also essential: both negative (e.g., injury,
sickness) and positive (e.g., high school graduation) outcomes should
be considered to ensure a balanced, constructive approach to health
policy development.

While some progress has been made in developing coherent and
testable theories of adolescent development that incorporate determinants, behavioural patterns, and both positive and negative

outcomes, this integrative aspect of adolescent health research is still young and lacks sufficient differentiation of risk-taking, health-promoting, and independence-seeking behaviours. Longitudinal studies are generally necessary to investigate these new developmental models, which have principally focused on child-to-adolescent transitions. Less attention has been given to developmental theories, which focus on adolescent-to-adult transitions.

The third objective of research, also relevant to policy development, is demonstration of intervention effectiveness. Research in this area is lagging in Canada as it properly depends on progress in the first two objectives and the subsequent development of coherent theory. Much of the literature on adolescent health interventions lacks adequate methodological rigour or follow-up. For example, meta-analyses of adolescent sexual health interventions have shown that they have no effect on key outcomes (DiCenso et al. 2002). We believe, however, that the real problem lies upstream, in insufficient outcome definition, specifically the need for a positive sexual health index as well as risk behaviours and STD/pregnancy outcomes. Meta-analyses may not be as useful for comparing behavioural interventions, due to their variation, as it is for pharmaceutical trials in which treatments are standardized and biological mechanisms are better understood.

To summarize, research can play a major role in health policy development if particular knowledge about health status, determinants, behaviours, and interventions can be assembled and interpreted.

AGE OF ADOLESCENCE

The definition of a child provided by the United Nations Convention on the Rights of the Child (UNCRC) represents a chronological-legal understanding of the child as "every human being below the age of eighteen years unless[,] under the law applicable to the child, majority is attained earlier" (United Nations 1989, Art. 1). In doing so, the period of adolescence is contained within the UN's general definition of a child, ignoring the reality of contemporary adolescence as well as its own policy on what constitutes youth (United Nations Secretariat 1999).

In general scientific usage, adolescence refers to the period beginning with puberty and ending with achieving the age of majority. The period of youth incorporates adolescence but extends beyond that into the young adult years. Confusion can occur since the start of puberty varies significantly among individuals, between genders, and across cultures. From a policy perspective, therefore, the timing and length of adolescence is variable. Childhood merges with adolescence and adolescence merges with, or extends into, the period of youth.

Our definition of adolescence is, consequently, more functional in nature: "Adolescence begins with the onset of physiologically normal puberty and ends when an adult identity and behaviour are accepted. This period of development corresponds roughly to the period between the ages of 10 and 19 years" (Canadian Pediatric Society Board of Directors 1994, reaffirmed in 2000). As such, adolescence is a period in the life cycle that has a biologic definition for its beginning but a socio-cultural definition for its end and that is of variable length.

Given the variable age of onset of puberty and the considerable variation between national and provincial legal markers of adult status – for example, age of voting, purchasing of tobacco products or alcohol, or obtaining a driver's licence – it is no wonder that policies and legislation with respect to adolescence are so fragmented and confusing in Canada. This book attempts to provide a basis for the development of more effective, and possibly inter-sectoral, policy for adolescents.

HEALTH GOALS FOR ADOLESCENTS

Adolescence is a time of flux and new beginnings in which young people grow physically, emotionally, intellectually, socially, and spiritually. This growth affects relationships with parents, peers, and romantic partners. Whereas earlier childhood development involves the complexity of genetics, health care, family structure, parenting, and early experiences, adolescent development adds the issues of emotional/sexual development, life planning, and participation in decision making and responsibility for one's own health.

The determinants-of-health approach and an emphasis on social factors, which generally assume passivity towards life circumstances and opportunities, can ignore the reality of more active behavioural aspects in adolescent health. Adolescence is a time of experimentation as young people begin to exert their independence. Risk-taking behaviour can be viewed as a vehicle for adolescent assertion of individuality and transition to adult status. Biologically based theories attribute risk-taking behaviour to genetic predispositions and hormonal changes mediated through pubertal timing. Psychological theories suggest that sensation-seeking, which reflects a need for varied, novel, and complex experiences, encourages a willingness to take physical and social risks. Risk-taking youth, for example, appear to think that they are invulnerable, that harm will never come to them. These perceptions and behaviours seldom occur in isolation but, rather, are often associated with peer group activities, some of which may lead to the development of unhealthy social norms.

Developmental models that recognize the transition phenomenon may be useful in understanding risk-taking during adolescence. Utilizing some of these models, Raphael (1996) presents a set of health goals for adolescents that includes:

(a) Making a successful transition from childhood to adulthood. Transition involves achieving independence, adjusting to sexual maturation, establishing cooperative relationships with peers, preparing for a meaningful vocation, achieving a set of basic beliefs and values, increasing autonomy and industry, and participating in community life (Conger 1991; Pederson et al. 1988);

(b) Coping and well-being, which involve making healthy choices related to nutrition, exercise, tobacco/alcohol/drug use, and sexuality;

(c) Absence of physical and mental illness as expressed by mortality and morbidity indicators: for example, physical disorders (such as obesity) and mental disorders (such as depression) (Offord, Boyle, and Racine 1989); and,

(d) Achieving healthy behaviours, which include health-enhancing and risk-avoidance behaviours, to address the concern that most adolescent health problems are due to injury and violence and risk-taking lifestyles that eventually affect health.

In this view, the health of adolescents, rather than being conceptualized as only the presence or absence of particular health problems, is understood as encompassing well-being or resiliency and the ability to cope with ups and downs in life and to learn from experience. The quality of the relationships that adolescents experience at school, at home, and in their communities determines how they feel about themselves and their prospects for the future as well as how they cope and adjust to challenges during their lives.

Regardless of which definition of health that academics and practitioners use, however, adolescents also create their own definitions. Health in adolescents, like learning, is an expressive and creative process connected to the values, beliefs, experiences, circumstances, and locations in which young people find themselves.

CURRENT DATA SETS AND MODELS OF DEVELOPMENT

We are fortunate in Canada to have a great deal of information on adolescent health issues, at least at the national level, much of which was presented in a report on the health of Canadians (Federal, Provincial, and Territorial Advisory Committee on Population Health 1999). We know, for example, that adolescents in Canada experience high rates of mental health problems, suicide, unintentional injuries (especially motor vehicle crashes), violence, and abuse. We also know that there are high rates of alcohol, tobacco, and other drug use as well as unsafe sex, and that some groups, such as economically and socially disadvantaged adolescents, experience these problems at significantly higher rates than others (King, Boyce, and King 1999; Health Canada 1999; Canadian Institute of Child Health 2000; Canadian Council on Social Development 2001).

The 2001–2002 Canadian instalment of the international Health Behaviour in School-Aged Children (HBSC) study (www.hbsc.org) provides an opportunity to explore some of the issues raised in this book in a single data set (Boyce 2004). This cross-sectional survey, administered every four years to approximately eleven thousand Canadian grade 6–10 students, has a wide focus on health of adolescents in school and, as such, can detect patterns between health and education sectoral variables and their change over time. The HBSC study is not designed to assess the impact of specific social, educational, and health system initiatives on the health of these young people but only to note whether outcomes and determinants of adolescent population health change over time.

From a population health perspective, the most powerful determinants of adolescent physical and emotional health that are evident from the 2002 HBSC survey are related to gender, family affluence, school conditions, and the influence of peers. Reinforcing evidence cited in this book, the factors that predict better adolescent health include greater wealth, good parent relationships, positive school experiences, and social integration with peers. The factors that predict poor adolescent health include early risk-taking, risk-taking by peers, and multiple risk-taking.

A serious limitation of existing Canadian cross-sectional studies of youth health, noted in this book by MacMillan et al., in Chapter 6, The Health and Well-being of Aboriginal Youths in Canada, is their failure to include or identify Aboriginal and other marginalized adolescents. These young people are often neglected for methodological reasons (i.e., insufficient numbers in specified geographic areas) without consideration for the possibility of over-sampling techniques. Another problem is in the failure to adequately include adolescents as stakeholders in these studies.

Once determinant and behavioural patterns are described, theories linking these with outcomes are possible. In the area of adolescence, with its inherent transitional nature, developmental theories that assume a process of change are appropriate. A number of developmental theories, both additive and predictive, have been posed that can be tested in longitudinal studies.

Simultaneous change models of development acknowledge that psychological, social, and biological changes in adolescence are often happening at the same time. *Cumulative events* models of development have a similar additive logic: the accumulation of disadvantage (e.g., poor economic status, poor home and community location, poor life chances via social networks, community values, and opportunities) can cause a gradient in outcomes (Simmons, Carlton-Ford, and Blyth 1987). An important consequence of the experience of simultaneous or cumulative change in the school and peer environment, in family roles, and pubertal development is that coping resources are overtaxed. Experiencing multiple and simultaneous events during early adolescence has been linked to depressed affect, lowered self-esteem, and a drop-off in school performance (Brooks-Gunn 1991; Petersen, Sarigiani, and Kennedy 1991; Simmons, Carlton-Ford, and Blyth 1987).

According to the *accentuation* model of development, puberty and other times of transition act to accentuate difficulties or to reinforce pre-existing behavioural patterns (Block 1982; Caspi and Moffitt 1991). In contrast to *personality theory*, which suggests that youth adapt to transitional events by reorganizing their behaviours and even their personalities, the accentuation model suggests that young people cope with stresses by assimilating existing patterns and cognitive structures into new risk-taking situations, mainly as a way of minimizing change. For example, early patterns of rough play among boys may lead to increased risk for injury in adolescent males.

The *latency* model of development suggests that an earlier event in a child's life, such as trauma, is predictive and may predispose him or her to negative outcomes during adolescence when stress occurs. Latency effects can be moderated in a negative (i.e., risk) direction through emotional insecurity or in a positive (i.e., protective) direction by effective parenting.

Similarly, the *trajectory* model (used by Rutter [1989] and Elder [1985]), which accounts for long-term influences from the social environment, suggests that the amount of time that a child associates with older peers at an early age will influence later risk-taking in drinking and sexual behaviours (Stattin and Magnusson 1990). A *pathway effect* is similar, although it focuses on social determinants, not behaviours. For example, status differences at birth, involving different levels of security, stability, and stimulation, may affect risk for poor school outcomes.

There does not yet appear to be a strong integrating thread through adolescent health research data. The plethora of theoretical approaches that are pertinent to adolescence – encompassing biological/hormonal, psychological, social, and economic fields – are not necessarily compatible. This is perhaps to be expected in a transitional state such as adolescence, and a more comprehensive understanding of adolescents and their health may be a distant goal.

SUCCESSES AND RESOURCES

Before suggesting possible solutions, we need to acknowledge our successes and the resources that we already have at our disposal. In this regard, there have been a number of recent encouraging developments in Canada. Among these are the establishment of research initiatives, the articulations of policy goals, the development of adolescent health action research projects, the establishment of research training opportunities, and researcher/policy-maker collaborations. All of these initiatives can make a contribution to the resolution of some of the issues discussed in this book and enhance the development of combined adolescent health policies in Canada.

For example, the Canadian Institutes for Health Research provide funding opportunities for the development of coordinated adolescent health research that could be directed at strengthening the evidence base, which, in turn, could be applied towards improved policy. CIHR funds are also available for training researchers in this field. The interest of the Federal, Provincial, and Territorial Advisory Committee on Population Health (1999) in national goals for healthy development of adolescents and young children could provide an impetus for the development of such policies and guidance regarding the specific information needed for coordinated adolescent health policies. Networks such as the Canadian Consortium for Health Promotion Research and the Canadian Adolescents at Risk Research Network provide infrastructures for mobilizing and developing research talent focusing on adolescent health issues and policies. Similarly, the networks for youth health research, such as the Centre of Excellence for Youth Engagement, provide vehicles for dialogue between researchers and practitioners on adolescent health policies. Finally, the production of this book has provided a forum in which debates regarding the link between evolving evidence-based frameworks and improved policies for adolescent health have occurred.

It is hoped that these debates will continue and expand as a result of the release and dissemination of this book so that Canada can indeed be a leader in the development of effective adolescent health policies. Building on these encouraging developments, there are a number of specific actions that might contribute to Canada's leadership in the development of such policies. These include the organization of workshops and conferences on coordinated adolescent health policies, the development of university and college courses (including distance learning courses) on the topic, the establishment of fellowships for research on adolescent health, and the development of a national agenda for adolescent health research. Through these means, and others suggested in these chapters, we can truly move ahead in our goal of improving the health of adolescents in Canada through the appropriate use of policy tools.

REFERENCES

Block, J. 1982. Assimilation, accommodation, and the dynamics of personality development. *Child Development* 53:281–95.

Boyce, William F. 2004. *Young People in Canada: Their Health and Well-Being*. Ottawa: Health Canada.

Brooks-Gunn, J. 1991. How stressful is the transition to adolescence in girls? In *Adolescent Stress: Causes and Consequences*, ed. M.E. Colten and S. Gore, 131–49. Hawthorne, NY: Aldine de Gruyter.

Canadian Council on Social Development (CCSD). 2001. *The Progress of Canada's Children*. 5th ed. Ottawa: CCSD.

Canadian Institute of Child Health (CICH). 2000. *The Health of Canada's Children: A CICH Profile*. 3rd ed. Ottawa: CICH.

Canadian Pediatric Society Board of Directors. 1994. Reference no. AM94–01. Ottawa: Canadian Pediatric Society.

Caspi, A., and T.E. Moffitt. 1991. Individual differences are accentuated during periods of social change: The sample case of girls at puberty. *Journal of Personality and Social Psychology* 61:157–68.

Conger, J.J. 1991. *Adolescence and Youth: Psychological Development in a Changing World*. 4th ed. New York: Harper Collins.

DiCenso, A., G. Guyatt, A. Willan, and L. Griffith. 2002. Interventions to reduce unintended pregnancies among adolescents: Systematic review of randomised controlled trials. *British Medical Journal* 324:1–9.

Elder, G.H., Jr. 1985. Perspectives on the life course. In *Life Course Dynamics: Trajectories and Transitions*, ed. G.H. Elder, Jr., pp. 23–49. Ithaca, NY: Cornell University Press.

Federal, Provincial, and Territorial Advisory Committee on Population Health. 1999. *Toward a Healthy Future: Second Report on the Health of Canadians*. Cat. no. H39–468–/1999E. Ottawa: Federal, Provincial, and Territorial Advisory Committee on Population Health.

Health Canada. 1999. *Healthy Development of Children and Youth*. Ottawa: Health Canada.

King, A.J.C., W.F. Boyce, and M. King. 1999. *Trends in the Health of Canadian Youth*. Cat. no. H39498/1999E. Ottawa: Health Canada.

McQueen, D., and L. Anderson. 2001. What counts as evidence? Issues and debates on evidence relevant to the evaluation of community health promotion programs. In *Evaluation in Health Promotion: Principles and Perspectives*, ed. I. Rootman, M. Goodstadt, B. Hyndman, D. McQueen, L. Potvin, J. Springett, and E. Ziglio, pp. 63–81. Copenhagen: European Regional Office of the World Health Organization.

Offord, D.R., M.H. Boyle, and Y.A. Racine. 1989. *Ontario Child Health Study: Summary of Initial Findings*. Toronto: Queen's Printer for Ontario.

Pederson, A., R. Edwards, M. Kelner, V.M. Marshall, and K.R. Allison. 1988. *Coordinating Healthy Public Policy: An Analytic Literature Review and Bibliography.* Ottawa: Minister of Supply and Services.

Petersen, A.C., P.A. Sarigiani, and R.E. Kennedy. 1991. Adolescent depression: Why more girls? *Journal of Youth and Adolescence* 20:247–71.

Raphael, D. 1996. The determinants of adolescent health: Evolving definitions, recent findings, and proposed research agenda. *Journal of Adolescent Health* 19(1):6–16.

Rutter, M. 1989. Pathways from childhood to adult life. *Journal of Child Psychology and Psychiatry* 30:23–51.

Simmons, R.G., S.L. Carlton-Ford, and D.A. Blyth. 1987. Predicting how a child will cope with the transition to junior high school. In *Biological-Psychosocial Interactions in Early Adolescence*, ed. R.M. Lerner and T.T. Foch, 325–75. Hillsdale, NJ: Eribaum.

Stattin, H., and D. Magnusson. 1990. *Paths through Life.* Vol. 2: *Pubertal Maturation in Female Development.* Hillsdale, NJ: Erlbaum.

Tones, K. 1997. Beyond the randomized controlled trial: A case for judicial review. *Health Education Research* 12(2):1–4.

United Nations Secretariat. 1999. *Youth Information Bulletin.* Vols. 1–2, nos. 98–9. New York: United Nations Secretariat.

United Nations. 1989. *Convention on the Rights of the Child.* Geneva: United Nations.

PART TWO

Key Examples of Adolescent Health Research and Policy

4

Socio-economic Status and the Health and Well-Being of Youths in Canada

LORI J. CURTIS

INTRODUCTION

The well-being of children was highlighted as a national priority in Canada in 1989, when an all-party motion of Parliament called for the elimination of child poverty in Canada by the year 2000. The following decade saw a number of changes to policies that affect families with children. In 1990, parental benefits were added to unemployment insurance (UI) benefits. The Canada Child Tax Benefit (CCTB) and the Earned Income Supplement (EIS) (also known as the Working Income Supplement, or WIS) were introduced in 1993. The year 1997 saw taxation changes on child support payments (such that the recipient was no longer required to pay tax on support and the payer no longer received a deduction for support), and the EIS was increased. The National Child Benefit was established in 1998 as a supplement to the CCTB and has increased over the years (Kamerman and Khan 1997; Jenson and Stroick 1999; Government of Canada 2006). Little evaluation of specific policy changes is available in the literature; however, analyses of the Child Tax Benefit find that benefits were shifted away from high-income families towards middle-class and moderately poor families, leaving the poorest families no better off (Kesselman 1993; Woolley et al. 1996). The focus of the policies has been overwhelmingly on assisting children rather than on assisting their parents.

Recent aggregate trends suggest that the national priority of improving the well-being of less fortunate children has remained elusive (Phipps 1999; Myles and Picot 2000). Phipps (1999) reports that poverty intensity (which consists of the combined measures of poverty rate, depth of poverty, and inequality) among those aged o to 18 years was actually higher in 1996 than in 1989. Crossley and Curtis (2006) point out that Canada's failure to meet this national priority "poses something of a puzzle, particularly in light of the success of other targeted anti-poverty agenda items, such as the drastic reduction in poverty among the senior population that had previously been achieved" (238).

Although broader definitions of health include mental, social, and spiritual health, well-being goes beyond this to include concepts such as standard of living, freedom, and justice that lead to one's overall happiness. There has been a plethora of research linking socio-economic status (SES) to health and well-being in both adult populations (e.g., Evans, Barer, and Marmor 1994) and child populations (e.g., Curtis et al. 2001; Vleminckx and Smeading 2001; Hertzman 2000; Heymann 2000; Keating and Hertzman 1999; Kohen, Hertzman, and Brooks-Gunn 1998; HRDC and Statistics Canada 1996). Socio-economic gradients, which describe the systematic increase seen in health and well-being outcomes as SES increases, are found across many outcomes used to measure adult and child health and well-being. Keating and Hertzman (1999) note that socio-economic gradients, similar to those reported in the general population health literature, were detected when studying child developmental outcomes like mathematics achievement, behavioural and school problems, general ability, mental health, and social adaptation.

Prior to 1996, the focus of research on the link between child health and well-being came from the Ontario Child Health Study (OCHS), which, at that time, was the only population-based longitudinal study of child health in Canada (Cadman et al. 1986; Offord et al. 1992). The OCHS surveyed children in 1983 and again in 1987 and, in the area of SES, found significant associations between low income and psychiatric disorder, social and educational functioning, and chronic physical health problems (Curtis et al. 2001; Lipman and Offord 1994; Lipman, Offord, and Boyle 1994; Cadman et al. 1986). Children living in lone-mother families were found to be at increased risk of a variety of psychiatric and academic problems (Curtis et al. 2001; Dooley et al. 1998; Lipman and Offord 1997; Dooley and Lipman 1996).

Dooley et al. (1998), among others, confirmed the OCHS results with findings from the National Longitudinal Survey of Children and Youth (NLSCY), a national sample of Canadian children released in 1996. The survey found a significant relationship between child psychosocial health and both lone-mother status and low income. The availability of these extensive data has allowed researchers to focus on many areas of child health and well-being in conjunction with SES, including, for example, the link between neighbourhood characteristics and health (Curtis et al. 2001; Kohen and Hertzman 1998), SES and readiness to learn (Kohen and Hertzman 1998), parenting style and child health (Burton, Phipps, and Curtis 2002; Chao and Willms 1998), and economic resources and children's health and success at school (Curtis and Phipps 2000).

To date, at least in the Canadian context, research and the resulting policy discussion have concentrated much more heavily on the relationship between SES and health among younger children than between SES and health among adolescents. Two explanations seem plausible. First, widely read documents such as *Growing Up in Canada* (HRDC and Statistics Canada 1996) and books such as *Developmental Health and the Wealth of Nations: Social, Biological, and Educational Dynamics* (Keating and Hertzman 1999) and *Labour Markets, Social Institutions, and the Future of Canada's Children* (Corak 1998), to list a few, have focused attention on the plight of poor children and placed an emphasis on early child development, the readiness of preschool children to learn, family functioning, and community factors affecting the long-term outcomes in young children. This is due in part to the focus on critical periods in early childhood development (see Duncan, Brooks-Gunn, and Maritato 1997 for a discussion of age groupings and the study of childhood poverty).

Another likely explanation has to do with the availability of data. The first wave of the OCHS in 1983 surveyed children (or their parents) from four to sixteen years, but, due to missing information for adolescents (non-response to survey questions), most analyses focused on children younger than twelve (see Curtis et al. 2001 for a description of the data). The NLSCY data, available to researchers via Statistics Canada's Research Data Centres (RDC), offer longitudinal information on children and youth. The availability of these data has facilitated a focus on children but seems to have done little to aid researchers in investigating similar relationships for the adolescents in our society.

The Health Behaviour in School-Aged Children (HBSC) survey is a notable exception to the data discussion. Studies coming out of the HBSC offer excellent information on the health status, health behaviours, and school and family environments of Canadian youths aged 11, 13, and 15 years (in grades 6, 8, and 10) and how these young people compare internationally (King et al. 1996; King and Coles 1992; King, Boyce, and King 1999; Mullan and Currie 2000; Currie et al. 2000). The overriding conclusion of the 1998 HBSC survey is that Canadian youths aged 11 to 15 years "appear to be well-adjusted in terms of physical and mental health, their relationships with their parents, peers, and school, and their health behaviours" (King, Boyce, and King 1999, 101). The findings also indicate, however, that youths experiencing poor relationships with family, peers, and/or teachers are far more likely to engage in health-risk behaviours, suffer from problems at school, and have poor health. Girls seem to do better at school, but they also have higher levels of stress and smoke more than do boys. The authors conclude that "more policy-directed research on the role of the family, school, and peer group in the health of youth is clearly required" (King, Boyce, and King 1999, 105).

Household income and poverty are not measured directly in the HBSC. Mullan and Currie (2000) provide a discussion on the difficulty and reliability of obtaining family income measures from youths who may not be privy to such information. The 1997/98 HBSC survey did include subjective questions on SES: for example, "How well off do you think your family is?" Children in grade 8 who answered "not well off" were substantially less likely (by between 35 % and 100 %) to (a) feel their parents understood them, (b) feel they belonged at their school, (c) report being very happy, and (d) abstain from marijuana use, when compared to those who reported their families as "well off" or "very well off" (King, Boyce, and King 1999). The 1998 cycle of the HBSC survey also included items in a family affluence scale (ownership of car/van, own bedroom, vacations) that measured disposable income or expenditures as a proxy for SES. Missing from these measures is an objective indicator of family income. Like other data sources mentioned previously, youths aged 16 and over were not included in the study.

This chapter attempts to fill these gaps and to document evidence on the relationship between SES (as measured by income status) and health, health behaviours, and the general well-being of youths aged twelve to nineteen, using data from cycle 3 (1998) of Canada's

National Population Health Survey (NPHS). We focus primarily on differences in health and well-being of youths in low-income households compared to those in higher-income households.

THE NATIONAL POPULATION HEALTH SURVEY

The National Population Health Survey includes a random sample of household residents of all ages in the ten Canadian provinces. It excludes individuals living on First Nations reserves; on Canadian Forces Bases; in the Yukon and Northwest Territories; and in some remote, northern areas of Ontario and Quebec; and those who are not residents in a household (i.e., the homeless). By excluding First Nations reserves and the homeless, the NPHS excludes some of the poorest populations in our society. Thus, any associations between poor outcomes and low income are likely to be an understatement of the true relationship.

The NPHS is a two-stage, stratified survey of households, and weights are used for all tabulations and calculations in this work. In all selected households, summary information is collected from a knowledgeable household member and then one member of the household is randomly selected for an in-depth interview. Thus, for the purposes of this chapter, we have good household information, such as income, home ownership, and so on, obtained from an individual in the household who is privy to such information. Personal health and health behaviours of youths twelve years of age and older are collected directly from the individual in the household (Statistics Canada 2000). This approach overcomes concerns about accuracy of information on parents or the household (such as income) as these data are not collected from youths (who may not have access to such information in the household), but they do answer questions on personal information.

The National Population Health Survey includes self-reported health status as well as information on personal and family characteristics, socio-economic status (SES), health behaviours, and labour force participation. The sample size of the in-depth health survey is 17,244 respondents, including 1,842 respondents between the ages of 10 and 19 years, which breaks down as 567 youths aged 12 to 14 and 926 aged 15 to 19 (Statistics Canada 2000). Approximately 350 children aged 10 and 11 years were interviewed, but many of

Lori J. Curtis

Table 4.1
Age distribution (%) of youths in Canada

	12–14 years	15–19 years
All	34.6	65.4
Females	33.9	66.1
Males	35.3	64.7

Source: Weighted estimates generated by the author using the 1998 National Population Health Survey (Statistics Canada. 2000. *National Population Health Survey, Cycle 3, 1998–1999*. Public Use Microdata Files Documentation. Ottawa: Statistics Canada.)

the relevant questions were only asked regarding individuals 12 years old and over. For this reason, the study focuses on this 12– to 19–year age group (1,493 individuals). Wherever possible, however, the tabulations were also performed including children ages 10 and over and the basic conclusions did not change. Table 4.1 indicates the age distribution of youths in Canada.

INCOME ADEQUACY AS A MEASURE OF
SOCIO-ECONOMIC STATUS

The distribution of youths across Canada is very similar to the population distribution. Almost 38% of youths live in Ontario, 23% in Quebec, 12% in British Columbia, 11% in Alberta, 10% in the Atlantic Provinces, and about 7% in the Prairies. In most provinces, these young people make up between 11% and 12% of the population, except for British Columbia and Newfoundland where 10% and 13.6% (respectively) of the population is between 12 and 19 years of age. Over 80% of those in this age group live in urban areas of Canada.

The focus of this chapter is on the relationship between SES and well-being among youths. Although data are presented on factors other than income that are related to SES, due to data limitations the main indicator of SES is an income adequacy measure. Income adequacy measures are based on total household income but take into account the number of individuals that rely on the income. Thus, an individual living in a family with two members and an annual household income of $40,000 per year is not included in the same category as someone from a family with the same household income but having six members. Table 4.2 presents the five income groups

Table 4.2
The five income groups and number of individuals dependent on the income

Lowest income group	< $10,000 with 1 to 4 persons AND < $15,000 with 5 or more persons
Lower-middle income group	$10,000 to $14,999 with 1 or 2 persons AND $10,000 to $19,999 with 3 or 4 persons AND $15,000 to $29,999 with 5 or more persons
Middle income group	$15,000 to $29,999 with 1 or 2 persons AND $20,000 to $39,999 with 3 or 4 persons AND $30,000 to $59,999 with 5 or more persons
Upper-middle income group	$30,000 to $59,999 with 1 or 2 persons AND $40,000 to $79,999 with 3 or 4 persons AND $60,000 to $79,999 with 5 or more persons
Highest income group	$60,000 or more with 1 or 2 persons AND $80,000 or more with 3 persons or more

Source: 1998 National Population Health Survey (Statistics Canada 2000, 34)

and the number of individuals dependent on the income from lowest to highest.

Although income adjusted for family size is a better indicator of economic circumstances than unadjusted income, we have no information on the intra-household division of the income and simply assume that it is shared equitably among household members. It is possible, of course, that this is not the case. There may be instances in which a member in a well-off family is "poor" due to unequal distribution of the resources (e.g., a wealthy couple in which one partner does not work and does not have access to equal shares of the income). It may also be the case that there is a member of a low-income household who does not appear to be poor (a plausible example is a poor lone mother who spends little on herself so that her child has the same clothes and toys as his/her peers). Unfortunately, these data do not contain any information on the allocation of income within the household.

Table 4.3 presents how the different age groups within the Canadian population fare in terms of economic well-being. The age groups are chosen to coincide, given the age categories available in these data, with ages that are generally discussed in research and policy documents. Children are designated as individuals under the age of 12 years. Youths are those between 12 and 19 years of age.

Table 4.3
Income adequacy categories by age group

	Child (under 12)	Youth (12–19)	Young adult (20–29)	Adult (30–59)	Senior (60 +)
All income groups	15.6	11.1	12.7	44.3	16.3
Lowest income group	3.2*	5.9	5.8 *	3.8*	3.8**
Lower-middle income group	13.2**	10.3	10.9	6.2*	16.4*
Middle income group	25.1	26.8	26.2*	22.2*	39.0*
Upper-middle income group	34.1	34.1	37.2	40.2*	29.7*
Highest income group	20.1	23.7	19.8**	27.6*	11.1**
p-value (null – income distribution same as youth)	0.021	not applicable	0.016	0	0
Low-income Group (Includes first two categories)	16.4	16.2	15.9	10.0*	20.2*

Source: Weighted estimates generated by the author using the 1998 National Population Health Survey (see Statistics Canada 2000 for more information on data)

* sig dif at 0.00, ** sig dif at 0.05

This division captures the age when individuals are searching for new freedoms outside the family environment, experiencing more independence with peers, through puberty to the end of high school. Those between the ages of 20 and 29 are labelled as young adults, an age when young people are making higher education, career, and early labour market choices. Those between the ages of 30 and 59 are classified as adults, and those 60 and over are seniors. The main comparisons focused on here are between youths, children, and seniors. As stated previously, recent research literature and policy initiatives have focused on the socio-economic status of children, particularly those living in poverty. Historically, the plight of seniors has received a great deal of attention and, as a consequence, policies were developed that reduced the poverty rates among this age group (Crossley and Curtis 2006; Phipps 1999). We now ask the question: are youths living in better circumstances than children and seniors?

The first row of data in Table 4.3 shows the distribution of age groups in the Canadian population. Not surprisingly, adults make up the largest group since adulthood covers the greatest age span. The other four groups are close in size, with seniors and children each accounting for about 16% of the population, youths making up 11%, and young adults about 13%. Both seniors and children make up a larger proportion of the population than do youths – another reason for the policy focus on these two age groups.

The left column of Table 4.3 lists the income adequacy categories available in the NPHS (introduced in Table 4.2), namely, lowest income, lower-middle income, middle income, upper-middle income, and highest income groups. Throughout the chapter, either these groups are used as specified or the first two groups (lowest income and lower-middle income) are combined to indicate a low-income group. It is noteworthy that, in Canada, there is no official poverty line and that measures put forth by Statistics Canada are low-income measures, not poverty measures. The rows in the table give the proportion of each age group that lies within the income adequacy categories. In all tables, the asterisks signify whether the percentage of individuals in the income category, by age group, is significantly different ($*p < 0.000$; $**p < 0.05$) than the percentage of youths in that income group. For example, 5.9% of youths live in lowest income households, while only 3.2% of children do so, and the difference is significant at the $p < 0.05$ level. The proportion of young adults in the lowest income category is the same as that for youths. Adults and seniors are identical, with 3.8% living in the worst economic circumstances.

A similar percentage of youths (10.3%) and young adults (10.9%) live in families classified as lower-middle income. Adults (6.2%) are significantly less likely to be in the lower-middle income category, while seniors (16.4%) and children (13.2%) are more likely to be classified as living in such households. The pattern is similar for the middle income category, except that children are as likely to be in this group as youths. The pattern changes, however, for those living in the best circumstances. About one-third of the three youngest groups, statistically identical, live in upper-middle income households. More adults (40%) and fewer seniors (30%) live under similar conditions. About 20% of children and young adults live in highest income households, with just under 24% of youths and just over 27% of adults having the best standard of living. Only 11% of seniors make it to the top category. The next row demonstrates that the income distributions of other age groups are not identical to those found in the youth group; in all cases the p-values are less than 0.05. Finally, the last row indicates the percentage of each age group living in low-income households, representing a combination of the households in the two lowest income categories. Approximately one out of every six children, youths, and young adults live in low-income households. Significantly fewer adults (10%) and more seniors (20%) live in the same circumstances.

In sum, the percentage of youths doing poorly, economically speaking, is about the same as for children but somewhat less than for seniors. Youths are more likely than seniors and children to be in the lowest income grouping, but, paradoxically they are also more likely than children and seniors to be in the best income category. Individuals in the adult group seem to have the best economic circumstances, with the smallest proportion living in low-income households and the highest proportion living in upper-income households.

Although the focus for most of the chapter is on income status, the next section gives an indication of how Canadian youths, specifically those aged 12 to 19, are faring vis-à-vis a variety of social and economic characteristics and how they compare across income categories.

ALTERNATIVE MEASURES OF ECONOMIC WELL-BEING

Income is not the only measure of economic well-being available in these data, nor is it the only measure of economic well-being of interest to policy-makers. Home ownership, number of bedrooms, and source of income may also be used as measures of material deprivation (Crossley and Curtis 2006; Curtis and Phipps 2000; Mullan and Currie 2000). Lone parenthood (Curtis 2001) and immigrant and visible minority status (Dunn and Dyck 2000) are a few examples of other measures used as indicators for material deprivation, longer-term poverty, or SES. Tables 4.4 and 4.5 demonstrate how Canadian youths, 12 to 19 years of age, are faring on these alternative measures of economic well-being. The tables also illustrate the correspondence between these measures and low-income status.

Home ownership may be used as an indicator of accumulated assets or wealth. Table 4.4 shows that approximately three-quarters of youths live in houses that are owned by a member of the household. The fraction falls drastically for youths in low-income

Table 4.4
Household characteristics by income status

	Percentage of all youth	Percentage of youth not in low-income households	Percentage of youth in low-income households
Home is owned by household member	76.5	85.2	31.7*
Number of bedrooms in house	3.31	3.4	2.8*
Child < 5 years lives in the home	7.2	6.7	9.5**
Child 6–11 years in the home	26.9	27.9	21.5**
Employment is the major source of income	90.1	95.4	61.6*
Transfers are the major source of income	7.9	3.2	32.8*
Major source of income listed as other	2	1.4	5.6*

Source: Weighted estimates generated by the author using the 1998 National Population Health Survey (see Statistics Canada 2000 for more information on data)

* sig dif at 0.00, ** sig dif at 0.05

households; slightly fewer than one-third of these youths live in accommodation that is owned by a family member. In households not considered to be low-income, 85% of youths live in a family-owned dwelling. Figure 4.1 indicates that the proportion of youths living in homes owned by a family member increases significantly across the income distribution. This is an excellent example of what researchers refer to as a gradient. The percentage of individuals who own their own home increases with each increase in income category.

The size of the home may also be a rough proxy for its value. The average number of bedrooms in youths' households is 3.3, with low-income households having 2.8 bedrooms while higher-income households have 3.4. Figure 4.2 also illustrates an income gradient in number of bedrooms across income categories, but the gradient is not as clear as in Figure 4.1. Thus, not only do significantly fewer low-income families with youths own their homes, they live on average in smaller homes.

Sources of income are very different across the income distribution. Ninety percent of all youth households list their major source of income as employment earnings; 95.4% of higher-income households claim the same, in contrast to only 62% of low-income households. Conversely, about one-third of low-income households list their main

Table 4.5
Individual characteristics by income status

	Percentage of all youth	Percentage of youth not in low-income households	Percentage of youth in low-income households
Female	47.7	46.7	53.0**
LIVING ARRANGEMENTS			
Youth lives with two parents	68.3	75.3	32.4*
Youth lives with single parent	16.8	12.9	36.9*
Youth is single (not living with parents)	4.1	1.4	18.1*
Youth is married	1	0.8	2.3**
Youth has a child	0.6	0.2	2.6*
Youth lives with child's other parent	0.3	0.2	0.6
Youth is a lone-parent	0.3	0	2.0*
Youth lives in other living arrangement	9.5	9.7	8.3
IMMIGRANT STATUS			
Youth is an immigrant	11.5	10.3	17.7**
Youth immigrated fewer than 4 years ago	31.2	26.5	48.5**
Youth immigrated 5–9 years ago	33.5	38.1	16.8**
Youth immigrated 10 years or more ago	34.5	34.4	34.7
YOUTH IS A VISIBLE MINORITY	15	13.1	20.3**
SCHOOL ATTENDANCE			
Youth attending school	87.1	89.6	74.4*
Youth (15–19) attending school	80.9	83.6	62.1*
Male youth (15–19) attending school	80.5	82.2	69.2*
Female youth (15–19) attending school	81.3	85.2	57.2*

Source: Weighted estimates generated by the author using the 1998 National Population Health Survey (see Statistics Canada 2000 for more information on data)

* sig dif at 0.00, ** sig dif at 0.0

source of income as transfers (e.g., social assistance), in contrast to only 3% of higher-income households. Figure 4.3 demonstrates the gradients in sources of earnings. Overall, Table 4.4 indicates that low income is strongly correlated with other measures of economic well-being and SES.

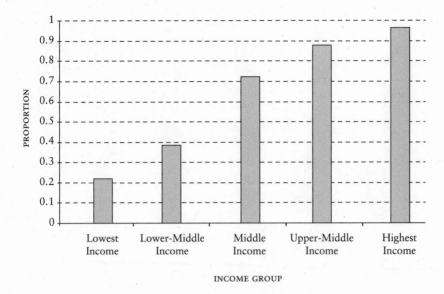

Figure 4.1
Proportion of youths living in a home that is owned by family member
by income status

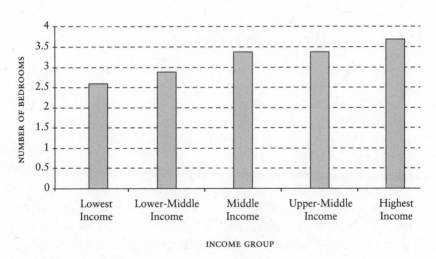

Figure 4.2
Number of bedrooms by income status

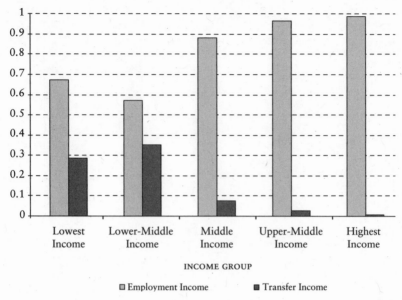

Figure 4.3
Proportion of youths living in households with employment or transfer earnings by income

Family Structure

Family status has also been closely linked to socio-economic status; many studies have shown that lone-mother families are much worse off socially and economically (e.g., Curtis 2001) than two-parent families. Table 4.5 indicates that this relationship holds for youths. The first row indicates that significantly more female youths live in low-income households. The second and third rows show that, although the vast majority of youths live with their parent(s), the proportion varies significantly by income status. Approximately two-thirds of all youths live in two-parent families; this proportion increases to 75% for youths not living in low-income households and decreases by half, to about one-third, for those living in low-income households. The pattern reverses for youths living in lone-parent households.

The differences are even more dramatic when looking at youths living on their own. Almost 6% of youths claim to be living on their own; 4% are single, 1% are married without children, and 0.6%

are living with their own children. The percentages are substantially different across the income divide. Just over 18% of youths who live in low-income circumstances report living on their own, 2.3% are married without children, and 2.6% have children. Of the youths who report having children and living in low-income households, almost all are lone parents. The small proportion of youths from higher-income groups who have children claim to be living with the child's other parent. Figures 4.4 and 4.5 demonstrate the distribution of household types across the income adequacy groups. Striking income gradients are seen across family types.

Ethnicity

Table 4.5 demonstrates the relationship between income status and immigrant/visible minority status among youths. Almost 12% of all youths are immigrants, but the percentage increases to about 18% of youths in low-income households. More low-income immigrant youths have been in the country fewer than four years compared to better-off youths. Based on self-reports by all youths over 12 years, 15% considered themselves to be members of a visible minority, but 20% of low-income youths fit that description.

School Attendance

Finally, almost 90% of youths from better-off households attend school, but only 75% of their low-income counterparts do. While males and females in the lowest income group are less likely to attend school than are those in higher-income groups, the picture is much more dramatic for females: approximately 70% of males in the lowest income group attend school, while only 40% of their female counterparts do. In other income categories, more females attend school than do males, but this was not tested statistically.

This statistic is even more startling when younger youths aged 12 to 14, who are legally compelled to attend school, are excluded from the analysis; Figure 4.6 shows the distribution of school attendance among youths aged 15 to 19 years by sex, as this is the age grouping available in the NPHS data. In most provinces, children must attend school until they are 16. It is also possible that youths in some provinces will have graduated by the age of 18. Eighty-four percent of older youths living in higher-income households attend

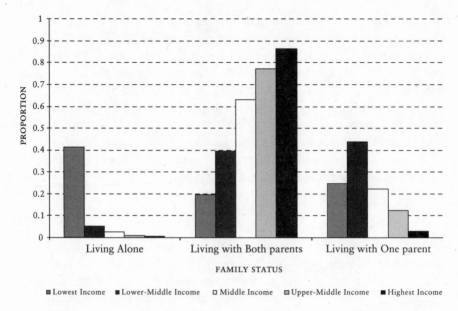

Figure 4.4
Family status by income group

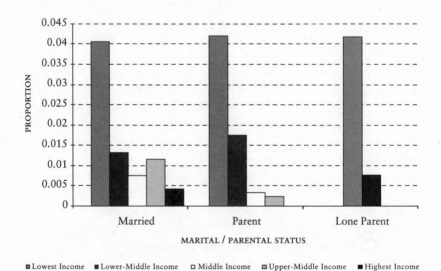

Figure 4.5
Marital/parental status by income group

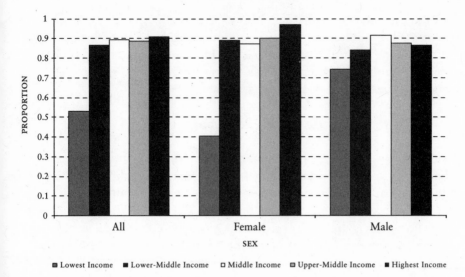

Figure 4.6
School attendance by income status and sex

school, compared to only 62% of older youths living in low-income households (Table 4.5). The picture is even bleaker for low-income females aged 15 to 19: only 57% attend school. Of note is the fact that only 37% of females in the lowest income category attend school on a full-time basis (Figure 4.6).

Education is certainly an important indicator of socio-economic status, and the percentage of low-income youths attending school is of concern due to the labour market consequences of poor educational outcomes. The extremely low school participation rate of low-income females is especially troubling because of the strong link between maternal education and child health.

The discussion, to this point, has centred on the socio-economic standing of youths in Canada. Youths are on average somewhat better off than seniors and about as well off as children; however, youths who live in low-income households are less likely to live in a home owned by a family member, and are more likely to live on their own, have children, and to be a lone parent than are those who live in higher-income circumstances. They are also more likely to be an immigrant or a member of a visible minority and less likely to attend school than are those who live in households that are classified as middle income or higher. Many, if not all, of the measures presented in Tables 4.3, 4.4, and 4.5 are considered to be broader determinants of health and well-being. Income status has also been tied to health behaviours and risk-taking for youths (Boyce 2004), and this is examined in the next section.

Health Behaviours

Health and risk-taking behaviours, such as smoking and exercise, have been closely linked to health and well-being in children, youths, and adults. The relationship between alcohol consumption and health is presently being debated, but it is acknowledged that alcohol consumption is linked to risk-taking behaviour (Boyce 2004). Table 4.6 presents information on the health and risk behaviours of youths by income status.

Few would argue with the fact that an active lifestyle reduces chance of heart disease, stroke, and a myriad of other health conditions, while smoking increases the likelihood of these problems. The first three rows of Table 4.6 give an impression of how active our youths are. Just over 43% of youths claim that they have a physically active lifestyle; 21% and 36% state they are moderately active or inactive, respectively. Youths living in low-income households are less likely to be physically active and more likely to be inactive than are better-off youths. Figure 4.7 displays activity levels across the entire income distribution. The higher-income groups are substantially more active than the lower-income groups. These patterns are similar across males and females (not shown).

First- and second-hand smoke is also directly related to health status. About one-third of all youths live in a household with a smoker. That proportion increases significantly to over 50% for low-income households. Approximately 27% of youths in low-income households smoke daily, a much higher percentage than for youths that are not in low-income households. Figure 4.8 demonstrates that the situation is even more dramatic for youths in the lowest income category, over 40% of whom smoke. Even more alarming is the fact that almost 50% of females in this income group smoke daily. For those who smoke regularly, the number of cigarettes consumed per day does not vary across income status; however, the age at which smoking began does vary. Poorer youths start smoking,

Table 4.6
Health behaviours and insurance status by income status

	Percentage of all youth	Percentage of youth not in low-income households	Percentage of youth in low-income households
PHYSICAL ACTIVITY			
Active lifestyle	43.2	44.8	34.8*
Moderately active lifestyle	21	21	21.1
Inactive lifestyle	35.7	34.1	44.1*
SMOKING BEHAVIOURS			
Smoker in household	36.8	33.8	52.4*
Daily smoker	14.6	12.2	26.7*
Occasional smoker	4.1	4.4	2.6
Smokes cigarettes	18.7	16.7	29.3*
Age started smoking	13.7	14	12.9*
Number cigarettes smoked daily	12.8	12.5	13.5
Ever smoked daily before	28.3	26.4	38.7**
ALCOHOL CONSUMPTION			
Ever drank alcohol	72	72.2	70.9
Drink alcohol regularly	31.6	31.9	30
Drink alcohol occasionally	21.3	20.7	24.5
PRIVATE INSURANCE STATUS			
Has drug insurance	76.4	79.9	58.5*
Has dental insurance	67.7	72.3	43.7*
Has optical insurance	58.5	62.9	36.2*
Has hospital insurance	62.4	68.5	31.8*

Source: Weighted estimates generated by the author using the 1998 National Population Health Survey (see Statistics Canada 2000 for more information on data)

* sig dif at 0.00, ** sig dif at 0.05

on average, at about 13 years of age – one year earlier than those who are better off.

The data in Table 4.6 indicate that there are not significant differences in alcohol consumption behaviour by low-income (i.e., the two lower income adequacy groups) versus non-low-income (i.e., the three higher income adequacy groups) cut-offs. Figure 4.9 illustrates, however, that youths living in the lowest income households drink regularly; and, once again, this is more pronounced for females. One-half of youths at the lower end of the income distribution drink alcohol regularly. Fifty-five percent of females and 41% of males

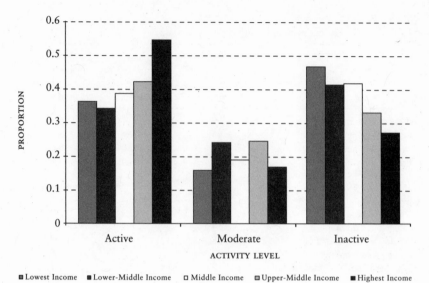

Figure 4.7
Activity status by income status

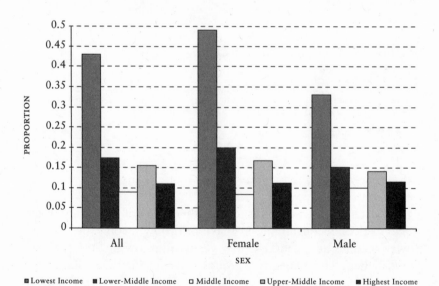

Figure 4.8
Proportion of youths who smoke daily by sex and income status

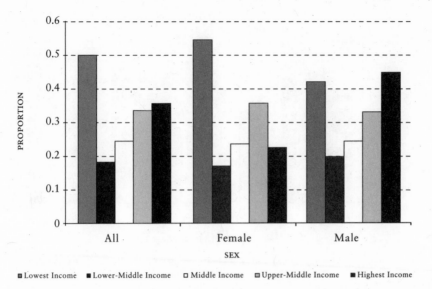

Figure 4.9
Proportion of youths who drink regularly by income status and sex

from the lowest income households drink regularly compared to 32% of all youths.

In sum, income status is clearly associated with health behaviours. Those with lower incomes are less likely to partake in health-creating behaviours and are more likely to participate in risky or unhealthy practices or to feel distressed.

Finally, having health insurance has been shown to be associated with health care utilization (Currie 1995). Public financing of health care in Canada has dwindled from 75% to 71% over the last few decades (CIHI 2000). The final rows of Table 4.6 demonstrate that youths who are economically disadvantaged are substantially less likely to be covered by private health insurance of any type, whether hospital, pharmaceutical, dental, or optical. Figure 4.7 demonstrates an income gradient across all of the insurance types. The plethora of research indicating that low-income status individuals have on average lower levels of health than do those with higher incomes, combined with the fact that the proportion of health-care costs covered by the public insurance system has been diminishing over the past three decades, makes this finding particularly worrisome.

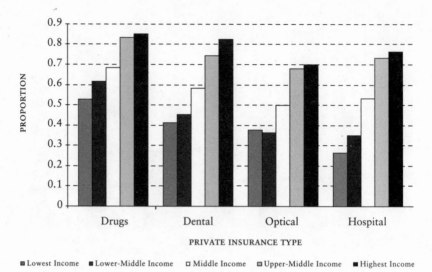

Figure 4.10
Proportion of youths covered by private insurance by insurance type and income status

Health Status

Overall, as indicated by Table 4.7, Canadian youths are healthy and happy. Over one-third of all youths report that they are in excellent health and almost 40% claim very good health status. When these two figures are combined, they reflect that over three-quarters of youths state that their health is very good or excellent. Furthermore, about one-fifth describe their health as good. Far fewer than 1% report they are in poor health, and about 2% declare fair health status; however, small numbers in the lowest health categories make comparisons unreliable. There are no significant differences across income categories for those youths who report health status at either end of the spectrum. When compared to those in higher-income categories, fewer youths in low-income households describe their health as very good and more describe their health as good.

About 12% of all youths claim they have asthma, while almost 17% of low-income individuals are asthmatic. On the other hand, about 20% of all individuals suffered an injury in the year before the survey; 16% of poorer youths compared to 22% of wealthier youths. This may reflect access on the part of wealthier youths to organized

Table 4.7
Health status indicators by income status

	Percentage of all youth	Percentage of youth not in low-income households	Percentage of youth in low-income households
Excellent health status	36.7	36.2	38.9
Very Good health status	44.2	45.8	36.1*
Good health status	17.5	16.2	24.1*
Fair health status	1.6	1.7	0.6
Poor health status	0.1	0	0.32
Has asthma	12.3	11.4	16.7**
Injuries in last year	21.4	22.4	15.8**
Vision problems in last year	24.3	23.5	28.9
Hearing problems in last year	0.2	0.2	0.1
Speech problems in last year	1	0.8	2.1**
Mobility problems in last year	0.2	0	0.2*
Cognition problems in last year	21.8	21.4	23.7
Pain problems in last year	2.7	2.2	5.4*
Emotional problems in last year	7.6	5.6	18.2*
Distress Index	3.4	3.3	4.0*

Source: Weighted estimates generated by the author using the 1998 National Population Health Survey (see Statistics Canada 2000 for more information on data)

* sig dif at 0.00, ** sig dif at 0.05

sports and vehicles. Fewer than one-quarter of youths from better-off households claimed to have problems with vision, while 29% of low-income youths claimed the same. The pattern is the same for problems with speech, mobility, cognition, pain, and emotions. In each case, youths living in low-income households claim to have more problems than those living in higher income households. Figure 4.11 characterizes the complete income distribution for the likelihood of suffering from vision, cognitive, and pain problems (the differences in hearing, speech, and mobility were too small to show on the chart). Once again, an income gradient is seen across the measures.

An income gradient is also seen for emotional problems for all youths and for females, but not for males (Figure 4.12). Low-income female youths experience the worst emotional health, with almost 60% reporting emotional problems; only 20% of males in the low-income group report problems.

In general, youths do well on the NPHS distress scale, which is derived from questions concerning whether or not the individual is

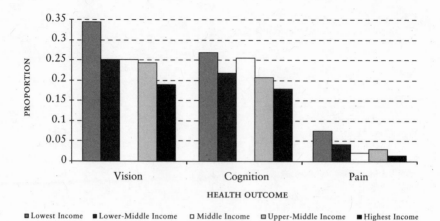

Figure 4.11
Proportion of youths with problems with vision, cognition, or pain by income status

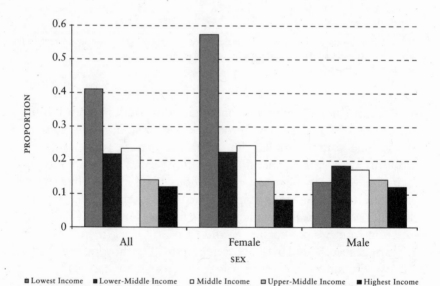

Figure 4.12
Proportion of youths reporting emotional problems by sex and income status

feeling sad, nervous, restless, hopeless, worthless, or that everything is an effort. The index is based on a subset of items from the Composite International Diagnostic Interview (CIDI). The score ranges from 0 to 24 and higher scores indicate more stress. As reflected in Table 4.7, low-income youths feel more distressed than do youths not in low-income households.

In sum, youths report being emotionally healthy; however, those in the lower-income groups are worse off than are those in higher-income groups. As well, females tend to fare worse than males.

DISCUSSION

Summary and Implications of Findings

To sum up briefly, when it comes to health, youths are faring relatively well. When investigating youths' health based on various measures, however, youths from low-income households do worse than other youths on the vast majority of measures. To put this in perspective, the relative proportions of youths and children living in low-income circumstances does not differ drastically, yet a higher proportion of youths live in the very poorest circumstances than do children or seniors (first row, Table 4.3). This finding is particularly disturbing considering that individuals on First Nations reserves and the homeless are not included in the study. Thus, the heavy focus by policy-makers and researchers on poverty among seniors and children but not among youths is puzzling.

Alternative measures of economic well-being are closely related to income status. Low-income families with youths are less likely to own their homes and more likely to have smaller homes. The income in such households is less likely to come from employment and more likely to come from income transfers – social assistance, for example – than in higher-income households. Poorer youths are much more likely to live with a lone parent, if they live with parents, and are more likely, on average, to live on their own or have children. If they have children themselves, youths from low-income households are more likely to be lone parents than are youths from better-off households. Youths from low-income households are also less likely to attend school than are those who live in households that are classified as middle income or higher. Young women living in low-income circumstances have the worst school attendance record.

A similar pattern is seen across youth health and risky behaviours and health status. Higher rates of inactivity, smoking, and alcohol consumption are seen in youths from low-income households. Females in the low-income categories do substantially worse than do males on many of the measures. Private health insurance coverage is particularly biased towards better-off youths. Canadian youths are, on average, very healthy, but, like the vast majority of other characteristics observed in this study, youths in lower-income circumstances fare less well than do those who have higher levels of income.

The simple associations presented in this chapter add to the growing literature that indicates that low income is related to poor health – in this case, for youth. Additionally, low income in youth is also related to low levels of education, lower levels of positive health behaviours, higher levels of negative health behaviours, less health insurance coverage, and lone parenthood. In turn, these characteristics are strongly related to poor health in children and adults (Curtis 2001; Curtis et al. 2001; Williamson and Fast 1998). If policy-makers are interested in improving the health status of the youth in our society, these factors must be addressed.

Phipps (1999) argues that we should be concerned about the health and well-being of children not only because, if treated well, they may grow into productive members of society who are ready and willing to support the next generation but also because they are important members of our society as children. The same can be said for youth. Youths are important members of our society: most are students, some are already in the labour force, and a few are already raising the next generation. Policy-makers should be interested in their economic circumstances now, due to strong relationships with health and well-being and because youths should be entitled to adequate living conditions as they grow up. The statistics presented in this chapter indicate that particular attention should be paid to females, aged 12 to 19, living in low-income households – the mothers of the next generation.

Recommendations for Policy-makers

The data presented in this chapter point to many mechanisms that policy-makers could use to improve the current and future well-being of our youth. Policies that promote a decline in smoking rates, excessive alcohol consumption, and teenage pregnancies and those that promote an increase in health insurance coverage, education, and incomes would all assist in improving the health and well-being of our youths. The following policy discussion focuses on three initiatives that are particularly relevant in today's environment of government funding cutbacks to our social safety net.

Much of the research in health indicates that policies should be directed at increasing income, education, and health insurance coverage, particularly of the poor; however, the current political agenda in most provinces is to cut income transfers and other programs historically associated with social assistance, like health insurance and education programs, in favour of increasing labour force participation. In general, individuals who are forced from the social assistance rolls end up in minimum-wage positions that offer no health insurance, paid sick/family leave, or avenues for advancement (Johnson and Corcoran 2002). This is not good news for youths living in households where the main source of income is social assistance. This is not an argument for policies designed to encourage individuals to rely on the state to support their families; rather, it is a call for incentives designed to offer individuals, who are able, the ability to earn incomes that will enable them to pay the fixed costs of work (like child and elder care, transportation, and health benefits) and maintain a reasonable standard of living after leaving social assistance.

Williamson and Fast (1998) show that the loss of health insurance, needed to cover medical necessities over and above those provided for by public health systems, for individuals who move from social assistance to paid work is a major determinant of lower levels of health for the working poor. Their research argues that health insurance should be provided to low-income workers, the unemployed, and students in order to guarantee access to necessary medical treatment, such as prescription drugs. This recommendation is particularly relevant as the proportion of health care covered by public insurance diminishes.

Individuals should be encouraged to obtain the tools required to avoid the necessity of social assistance. Programs directed at enabling youths to remain in the educational system, leading to increases in labour market outcomes and thus better incomes (and health insurance coverage), would alleviate the necessity of social assistance for many youths. Increasing education could also lead directly to better health-related habits (less smoking and more active lifestyles) and better health for youths (especially female) and their future children (as maternal health is strongly associated with child health). In a study, the present author found that higher income and education for mothers had much greater associations with their improved health than did decreasing their smoking by half or increasing their activity levels (Curtis 2001). Few would argue that funding programs that could decrease the number of cigarettes smoked or increase activity rates would not be worthwhile activities when it came to increasing population health status; however, the extent that these child-based results can be generalized to the youth population, increased education and thus income could have greater effects in changing health habits. Attempts to change lifestyle factors by themselves may be limited in scope. There may be little hope of improving lifestyle factors if the basic problems of poverty and poor education are not first addressed. Higher levels of income and education could lead both directly and indirectly, via improved lifestyles, to improved health and well-being.

Income transfers, similar to those available in countries like Norway, should be available for families, particularly lone-parent families, who are unable to participate in the labour force due to child care responsibilities (see for example Curtis and Phipps 2004). The income transfers in Norway are substantial and are not designed to be punitive or to cause societal stigma for families who receive them. The policies are directed at supporting families under a value system that holds that parents are the guardians of the next generation and that the entire society should be responsible for raising future generations.

This chapter also indicates that research into the health and well-being of youths should be a much higher priority. In particular, there should be an emphasis placed on understanding the situations of females from lower-income households. This is not to suggest that research into child health and well-being should be emphasized less but, rather, that youth health and well-being should also be a research and policy focus. In some circumstances, youths may be even more vulnerable than children; they may no longer reside with parents who can offer assistance and support on a day-to-day basis. More policy-relevant research is needed for this age group, particularly when familiar policies, such as anti-smoking and anti-drinking campaigns, do not seem to affect the lives of youths, in particular female youths.

REFERENCES

Boyce, William F. 2004. *Young People in Canada: Their Health and Well-being*. Cat no. H39–498/2004E. Ottawa: Health Canada.

Brooks-Gunn, Jeanne, Greg Duncan, and Nancy Maritato. 1997. Poor families, poor outcomes: The well-being of children and youth. In *Consequences of Growing Up Poor*, ed. G. Duncan and J. Brooks-Gunn, 1–17. New York: Russell Sage Foundation.

Burton, Peter, Shelley A. Phipps, and Lori J. Curtis. 2002. All in the family: A simultaneous model of parenting style and child conduct. *American Economic Review, Papers and Proceedings* 92(2):368–72.

Cadman, D., M.H. Boyle, D.R. Offord, P. Szatmari, N.I. Rae-Grant, and J. Crawford. 1986. Chronic illness and functional limitation in Ontario children: Findings of the Ontario Child Health Study. *Canadian Medical Association Journal* 135:761–7.

Canadian Institute for Health Information (CIHI). 2000. *National Health Expenditure Trends, 1975–2000*. National Health Expenditure Database. Ottawa: CIHI.

Chao, Ruth K., and J. Douglas Willms. 1998. Do parenting practices make a difference? Human Resources Development Canada Working Paper w-98-32Es.

Corak, Miles, ed. 1998. *Labour Markets, Social Institutions, and the Future of Canada's Children*. Ottawa: Statistics Canada.

Crossley, Thomas F., and Lori J. Curtis. 2006. Child poverty in Canada. *Review of Income and Wealth* 52(2):237–60.

Currie, C., K. Hurrelman, W. Settertobulte, R. Smith, and J. Todd. 2000. *Health and Health Behaviour among Young People*. Copenhagen: World Health Organization Regional Office for Europe.

Currie, Janet. 1995. Socio-economic status and child health: Does public health insurance narrow the gap? *Scandinavian Journal of Economics* 97(4):603–20.

Curtis, Lori J. 2001. Lone motherhood and health status. *Canadian Public Policy* 27(3):335–56.

Curtis, L.J., M.D. Dooley, E.L. Lipman, and D.H. Feeny. 2001. The role of permanent income and family structure in the determination of child health in Canada. *Journal of Health Economics* 10:287–302.

Curtis, L.J., and S.A. Phipps. 2000. Economic resources and children's health and success at school: An analysis with the National Longitudinal Survey of Children and Youth. Human Resources and Development Canada Working Paper.

Curtis, Lori J. and Shelley A. Phipps. 2004. Social transfers and the health status of mothers in Norway and Canada. *Social Science and Medicine* 58(12):2499–507.

Dooley, M.D., Lori J. Curtis, Ellen Lipman, and David Feeny. 1998. Child behaviour problems, poor school performance, and social problems: The roles of family structure and low income in Cycle One of the National Longitudinal Survey of Children and Youth. In *Labour Markets, Social Institutions, and the Future of Canada's Children*, ed. Miles Corak, 107–27. Ottawa: Statistics Canada.

Dooley, M.D., and Ellen Lipman. 1996. Child psychiatric disorders and poor school performance: The roles of family type, maternal market work, and low income. In *Towards the XXIst Century: Emerging Sociodemographic Trends and Policy Issues in Canada*, 135–143. Proceedings of a Symposium of the Federation of Canadian Demographers, Saint Paul University/Université Saint-Paul. Ottawa: Federation of Canadian Demographers.

Dunn, James R., and I. Dyck. 2000. Social determinants of health in Canada's immigrant population: Results from the National Population Health Survey. *Social Science and Medicine* 51(11):1573–93.

Evans, Robert G., Morris L. Barer, and Theodore R. Marmor, eds. 1994. *Why Are Some People Healthy and Others Not? The Determinants of Health of Populations*. New York: Aldine de Gruyter.

Government of Canada. 2006. *The National Child Benefit*. Ottawa: Government of Canada. http://www.nationalchildbenefit.ca/home_e. html. Retrieved 10 September 2008.

Hertzman, Clyde. 2000. The case for an early child development strategy. *ISUMA: Canadian Journal of Policy Research* 1(2):11–18.

Heymann, Jody. 2000. *The Widening Gap*. New York: Basic Books.

Human Resources Development Canada (HRDC) and Statistics Canada. 1996. *Growing Up in Canada: National Longitudinal Survey of Children and Youth*. Ottawa: Statistics Canada.

Jenson, Jane, and Sharon Stroick. 1999. *A Policy Blueprint for Canada's Children*. Reflexion Research Report No. 3. Ottawa: Canadian Policy Research Network.

Johnson, R., and M. Corcoran. 2002. *Welfare Recipients' Road to Economic Self-Sufficiency: Job Quality and Job Transition Patterns Post-PRWORA*. Ann Arbor: University of Michigan. http://www.ford-school.umich.edu/research/poverty/pdf/JPAMFIN1.pdf. Retrieved 1 August 2006.

Kamerman, Sheila B., and Alfred J. Kahn. 1997. *Family Change and Family Policies in Great Britain, Canada, New Zealand, and the United States.* New York: Oxford University Press.

Keating, D.P., and C. Hertzman, eds. 1999. *Developmental Health and the Wealth of Nations: Social, Biological, and Educational Dynamics.* New York: Guilford Press.

Kesselman, Jonathan. 1993. The Child Tax Benefit: Simple, fair, responsive? *Canadian Public Policy* 19(June):109–32.

King, A.J.C., W.F. Boyce, and M. King. 1999. *Trends in the Health of Canadian Youth.* Ottawa: Health Canada.

King, A.J.C., and B.J. Coles. 1992. *The Health of Canada's Youth: Views and Behaviours of 11–, 13–, and 15–year-olds from 11 Countries.* Ottawa: Health and Welfare Canada.

King, A.J.C., B. Wold, C. Tudor-Smith, and Y. Harel. 1996. The health of youth: A cross-national survey. WHO Regional Publication, European Series No. 69.

Kohen, Dafna, and Clyde Hertzman. 1998. Affluent neighbourhoods and school readiness. Working Paper No. w-98–15Es. Ottawa: Human Resources Development Canada.

Kohen, Dafna, C. Hertzman, and J. Brooks-Gunn. 1998. Neighbourhood influences on children's school readiness. Working Paper No. w-98–15E. Ottawa: Strategic Policy, Applied Research Branch, Human Resources Development Canada.

Lipman, E.L., and D.R. Offord. 1994. Disadvantaged children. In *The Canadian Guide to Clinical Preventive Health Care,* 356–68. Cat. no. H21–117/1994E. Ottawa: Canadian Task Force on the Periodic Health Examination, Minister of Supply and Services Canada.

– 1997. Psychosocial morbidity among poor children in Ontario. In *Consequences of Growing Up Poor,* ed. G. Duncan and J. Brooks-Gunn, 239–87. New York: Russell Sage Foundation.

Lipman, E.L., D.R. Offord, and M.H. Boyle. 1994. Economic disadvantage and child psychosocial morbidity. *Canadian Medical Association Journal* 151:431–7.

Mullan, Elaine, and Candace Currie. 2000. Socio-economic inequalities in adolescent health. In *Health and Health Behaviour in Young People,* ed. Candace Currie, Klaus Hurrelman, Wolfgang Settertobulte, Rebecca Smith, and Joanna Todd, 65–72. Copenhagen: World Health Organization.

Lori J. Curtis

Myles, John, and Garnet Picot. 2000. Poverty indices and policy analysis. *Review of Income and Wealth* 46(2):161–79.

Offord, D.R., M.H. Boyle, Y.A. Racine, J.E. Fleming, D.T. Cadman, H.M. Blum, C. Byrne, P. Links, E.L. Lipman, H.L. MacMillan, M.N. Sanford, P. Szatmari, H. Thomas, and C.A. Woodward. 1992. Outcome, prognosis, and risk in a longitudinal follow-up study. *Journal of the American Academy of Child and Adolescent Psychiatry* 31:916–23.

Phipps, Shelley. 1998. *An International Comparison of Policies and Outcomes for Young Children.* Reflexion Research Report No. 5. Ottawa: Canadian Policy Research Network 135:761–7.

– 1999. Economics and the well-being of Canadian children. *Canadian Journal of Economics* 32(5):1135–63.

Statistics Canada. 2000. *National Population Health Survey, Cycle 3, 1998–1999.* Public Use Microdata Files Documentation. Ottawa: Statistics Canada.

Vleminckx, K., and T.M. Smeading, eds. 2001. *Child Well-Being, Child Poverty, and Child Policy in Modern Nations.* Bristol: Policy Press.

Williamson, D.L., and J.E. Fast. 1998. Poverty status, health behaviours, and health implications for social assistance policy. *Canadian Public Policy* 24(1):1–25.

Woolley, Frances, Arndt Vermaeten, and Judith Madill. 1996. Ending universality: The case of child benefits. *Canadian Public Policy* 22(1):24–39.

5

Health Promotion
through School Improvement

ANDY ANDERSON AND WILLIAM BOYCE

Health promotion is the process of enabling people to increase control over and improve their health. To reach a state of complete physical, mental, and social well-being, an individual or group must be able to identify and realize aspirations, satisfy needs, and change the environment or cope with it. Health is therefore seen as a resource for everyday life, not the final objective of living. Health is a positive concept that emphasizes social and personal resources as well as physical capacities. Therefore, health promotion is not just the responsibility of the health sector; it goes beyond developing healthy lifestyles to achieving well-being in all settings (World Health Organization 1986).

The variables that interact with and work to determine adolescent health are numerous and are discussed throughout this book. In this chapter, we focus on some of the factors that create capacity for health in school settings. The main tasks of education are to facilitate identity development and teach how to participate in society (through knowledge, skills, and behaviour) (ten Dam 2002). A focus on health in schools is intended to support these goals and is achieved not just through an appropriate health curriculum but in a myriad of ways that involve students, parents, teachers, and administrators. A holistic approach to health promotion in schools leads not only to healthier students but also to improved schools and educational effectiveness. The achievement of educational goals through addressing health issues is the main strategy of the health-promoting school movement (St Leger 2001; Anderson 1999, 2000).

The development of effective health promotion practices in schools requires a clear understanding of the capabilities and limitations of schools in generating health. It is important for policy-makers to understand that, in order to be successful, efforts to improve adolescent health through school programs must be accompanied by programs and supports at all levels of society. Schools can only do so much, and they are but one setting in which adolescents learn health practices. Schools are also key components of communities and can contribute to social capital opportunities for youth.

A number of key policy elements exist for the effective implementation of health promotion specifically in schools, and we discuss these in this chapter. First, a policy framework based on the goals of "health-promoting schools" (to be described later) needs to be deeply embedded in ministerial, board, and local school policy development. Second, a formal health education curriculum that supports health-promoting activities and concepts in all other parts of the curriculum is required. Third, the participation of parents, students, teachers, school principals, and the local health sector needs to be strengthened in health-promoting activities.

SCHOOL AS A UNIQUE SETTING FOR HEALTH PROMOTION

Schools are a microcosm of society and youth culture (Smith and Lusthaus 1994). Canadian schools form the "workplace" of 20% of the Canadian population, including 5,000,000 students and over 400,000 employees. Another 30% of the population – parents – have a direct stake in schools through their children (Canadian Association for School Health 1991). School thus represents a unique and significant setting through which adolescent health promotion can be achieved.

The school years are a time of rapid individual and social development, during which many elements of attitude and behaviour, health literacy, and skills which impact on future health are still forming. Children's health behaviours and their views of themselves have been shown to be related to their lives in school (Rudd and Walsh 1993; Resnick, Harris, and Blum 1993). Experiences at school have been shown to have a profound influence on the social and emotional development of young people (Marx, Wooley, and Northrop 1998).

The mutually supportive relationship between education and health has been well documented. Healthy children learn better (Allensworth 1993; Lavin, Shapiro, and Weill 1992), while children who are sick, tired, and afraid have trouble learning (Kolbe 1985, 1986; Anderson and Piran 2001). Healthy children miss fewer days of school, cope better with adversity and transitions in their lives, and get along better with their peers (Jessor 1993; Anderson et al. 1999). Just as health exerts a powerful influence on children's ability to learn, so educational achievement is an important determinant of health. Students who have adjusted well to school are more likely to enjoy school life, engage in postsecondary studies, "have good relationships with their parents ... be healthy and happy, and ... avoid health-risk behaviours" (King, Boyce, and King 1999, xiii). In the long term, a good education enables people to attain fulfilling and stable employment and, as a result, to enjoy higher standards of living that contribute to health (e.g., housing, health care, and leisure and recreational pursuits) (Stephens and Fowler Graham 1993).

School is in many instances a safe haven for adolescents. As poverty, family conflict, drugs, neighbourhood violence, prostitution, and toxic environments increasingly plague many communities (Glazier et al. 2000; O'Loughlin et al. 1999), a greater percentage of youths become reliant on the school as the only stable influence in their lives (Dryfoos 1990; Valpy 1993). School connectedness, according to Resnick, Harris, and Blum (1993), is the most salient protective factor for both girls and boys against acting-out behaviours, and it is second in protective importance after family connectedness for "quietly disturbing behaviours" such as bulimia and suicide.

On the negative end of the spectrum, school can also be a place where youths are exposed to a number of health-compromising behaviours, such as smoking, alcohol and drug use, unwanted or high-risk sexual activity, racism, and violence. Some adolescents experience school as a threatening place where unreasonably high expectations create an environment of criticism and exclusion. As a result, some youths gradually disengage from school life. Recent research has demonstrated that a process of disengagement from school typically leads to involvement with other youths who share similar feelings and values and who ultimately engage in health-risk behaviours together (Connop and King 1999).

It is evident that school and education experiences have significant and direct impacts on the short- and long-term health status and behaviour of adolescents. Likewise, student health status has a great impact on ability to learn and to experience positive, successful school lives. The school is the one setting in which most adolescents can be reached – irrespective of their socio-economic status, ethnicity, or location – and through which their health concerns can potentially be addressed (St. Leger 2001). School health is, however, much more than a course of study. Influences on health are also evident in the curricular, extracurricular, social, and civic elements of school. School structure and operational procedures, curricula and teaching methods, and the manner in which student progress is assessed can have direct effects on students' self-esteem, educational outlooks, and achievement levels, which are themselves key determinants of adolescent health (Rutter 1979; Sammons, Hillman, and Mortimore 1995). The overall policy problem lies in how to facilitate a mutually supportive relationship between health and education in order to promote youth health in its full complexity.

POLICY FRAMEWORKS
FOR HEALTH-PROMOTING SCHOOLS

There have been three phases of evolution in the education and health partnership as it relates to schools: schools as convenient venues, schools as institutions, and schools as educational institutions (Nutbeam 2002). In "schools as convenient venues," schools were seen as an important point of access to young people for classroom-based educational programs directed towards risk behaviours (e.g., smoking, drug use, sexual activity). In "schools as institutions," classroom-based interventions were seen as unsustainable without various forms of institutional support. The influence of the hidden curriculum, school organization, and climate on classroom-based work was recognized. In the current phase, "schools as educational institutions," it is now recognized that schools are not merely convenient institutions for health promotion. It is understood that curriculum time for health education is limited, specialist teacher training and support requires time and resources, and policy and environmental change in schools is difficult to implement and sustain.

The complex relationship between education and health, and particularly its multisectoral and cross-jurisdictional nature, requires a broadly accepted policy framework in order to realize its potential. Although much has been written about health promotion in school settings, there is very little research that describes how health-promoting schools are created and the educational and health outcomes of such an initiative (St Leger and Nutbeam 2000).

In 1996, the Australian National Health and Medical Research Council (NHMRC) Health Advancement Standing Committee reviewed the literature concerning health promotion in schools. The Committee found that the interaction between schools and young people, and the overall experience of attending school, presented unique opportunities for health promotion. It concluded that programs that were comprehensive, integrated, and holistic, and that embraced aspects across the curriculum, the environment, and the community, were more likely to lead to advancement in the health of school children.

The concept of "health-promoting schools" is useful at the ministerial, board, and local school levels (NHMRC Health Advancement Standing Committee 1996). The concept takes a holistic view of health promotion and sees it as a strategy for:

(a) improving working conditions for teachers and learners;
(b) increasing opportunities for both teachers and students to participate in the changes that matter most to them;
(c) broadening and deepening student involvement in assessment activities, action planning, decision making, and resource mobilization; and
(d) engaging partners in the school improvement process.

The European Network of Health Promoting Schools (ENHPS) and Comprehensive School Health (CSH) are two models of health promotion that have been used in schools. Both offer conceptual and organizational frameworks for ministries of education that adhere to the key principles of health promotion and school improvement listed above.

EUROPEAN NETWORK OF HEALTH PROMOTING SCHOOLS (ENHPS)

The European Network of Health Promoting Schools (ENHPS) was pilot-tested in 1991 in Hungary, the Czech Republic, Slovakia, and Poland. It was formally launched in 1992 as a collaborative project of the European Commission, the Council of Europe, and the World Health Organization (WHO) Regional Office for Europe. Since then it has expanded rapidly, with over forty countries participating in the network through health-promoting school projects intended to influence the health of about 400,000 young people in over five thousand schools.

Countries wishing to join the network are required to have support from both their ministry of education and ministry of health. A national coordinator must be appointed and ten schools must be designated that are willing and able to collaborate. Participating schools work together and each is expected to meet the following requirements:

(a) develop a three-year project plan;
(b) form a school project team and prioritize project activities;
(c) implement projects to tackle issues of both local and European relevance;
(d) implement activities that promote the health of young people and foster a spirit of collective responsibility for personal and community health as well as maximize the project's visibility and credibility; and
(e) facilitate the evaluation and dissemination of results (Anderson and Piran 2001).

Ten principles guide the practice of health promotion in ENHPS, and these are listed in Table 5.1. These include the underlying values and goals of democracy, equity, and empowerment. ENHPS creates structures and relationships in schools based on these values, recognizing that these must be in place to enable each student to achieve optimal health. Other principles include the recognition that social and physical factors in the school environment must be addressed in health promotion efforts. The ENHPS has proven to be an effective and progressive framework for the development of health promotion programs and policy in European schools (Anderson and Piran 2001).

COMPREHENSIVE SCHOOL HEALTH (CSH)

In Canada, Comprehensive School Health as a model for health promotion has received acceptance at various levels. CSH has been described as a broad spectrum of programs, policies, activities, and services that take place in schools and neighbourhoods (CASH 1991). The model was originally developed by Health Canada, the Canadian Association of School Health, and educational bodies across the

Table 5.1
Ten principles of the European network of health promoting schools

Principle	Description
1) Democracy	Connect educational experiences and learning to people's lives, issues, and circumstances; explore alternative perspectives; engage students in applying what they are learning to improvements in society; contribute ideas and insights to debate and understanding
2) Equity	Endeavour to make schools free from oppression, fear, and ridicule; provide equal access for all to the full range of educational opportunities; foster the emotional and social development of every individual; enable each student to attain his/her full potential free from discrimination
3) Empowerment	Improve young people's abilities to take action, cope, and generate change; link young people's empowerment to their visions and ideas and enable them to take actions that improve their lives and living conditions
4) School environment	Acknowledge both physical and social environments as crucial factors in promoting and sustaining health; ensure the formulation and monitoring of health and safety measures and the introduction of appropriate management structures
5) Curriculum	Provide opportunities for young people to gain knowledge and insight and to acquire essential life skills; enable the curriculum to act as an inspiration for teachers and others working in the schools and a stimulus for their own personal and professional development
6) Teacher training	Acknowledge it as an investment in health as well as education, in which teaching is seen as a learning profession and professional learning experiences result in high quality teachers and learning experiences for students
7) Measuring success	View as a means of support and empowerment and an integral part of the teaching/learning process
8) Collaboration	Make a central part of the strategic planning process
9) Communities	Give a vital role to play in leading, supporting, and re-enforcing the concept of school health promotion
10) Sustainability	Structure and support plans and action for long-term and continuous renewal, such that health-promoting schools are seen as "here to stay"

Source: (Anderson and Piran 2001, 4)

country. Policies, programs, services, and activities delivered using comprehensive approaches are the responsibility of those concerned with the education and health of children and youth, including families, professionals, institutions, agencies, governments, and other organizations and even young people themselves. Participation in CSH is multisectoral, including education, health, social services, law enforcement, business, voluntary groups, labour, and governments at all levels.

The CSH model suggests that health promotion practices in schools are comprehensive when:

(a) instruction about health includes all areas of the health curriculum – nutrition, physical activity, safety and injury prevention, substance abuse prevention, growth and development (i.e., sexual health education);
(b) instruction includes study of both individual and environmental factors that affect decisions for health, in addition to coping and communication skills;
(c) social support from parents, peers, policy-makers, staff, local media, and the community are aligned with educational programs and services;
(d) other support services for children, youth, and families (psychological assessment and counselling, provision of special programs for persons with disabilities) are coordinated with school resources and personnel; and
(e) the school environment reflects and nurtures opportunities for optimal learning. (McCall 1999)

Some examples of Comprehensive School Health in action are listed in Table 5.2.

INTERNATIONAL SUPPORT
FOR ENHPS AND CSH

Both ENHPS and CSH suggest that health promotion is situated within the wider context of educational improvement and overall improvements in society. This approach is supported and reflected in the approaches and/or official stances of international organizations such as the World Health Organization and the United Nations. The World Health Organization describes a health-promoting school as

Table 5.2
Comprehensive school health in action

Area	Features
Instruction	• a K-12 health/personal development curriculum • a physical education and family studies curriculum • effective teacher in-service and pre-service training • relevant high quality teaching/learning materials • appropriate teaching methods • informal learning with peers and parents
Social support	• peer helper and support programs • adult role models and mentors • positive school climate • healthy public policy from school boards, boards of health, and social agencies • family/parent involvement • formal needs assessment and planning
Support services	• appropriate health and social services for children/adolescents and families • school guidance services • student services • support for inter-agency, inter-ministry, and inter-disciplinary co-operation • an integrated web of services offering appraisals, referrals, treatment, and follow-up • in-service and pre-service training for nurses and other professionals
Physical environment	• safety and accident prevention measures in the school and playgrounds • healthy food choices and meal programs where needed • smoke-free policy • alcohol- and drug-free policies • prohibition of harassment and discrimination

Source: McCall, D. 1999. Comprehensive school health: Help for teachers from the community. *Canadian Association for Health, Physical Education, Recreation, and Dance* 65(1):4–9.

a system that constantly strengthens its capacity as a healthy setting for living, learning, and working (WHO 1995). It focuses on creating health and preventing major causes of death, disease, and disability by helping members of the school community care for themselves, make decisions, have control over the circumstances that affect their health, and create environments that are conducive to health.

The United Nations Convention on the Rights of the Child, which has near universal ratification by countries from all parts of the globe, also supports the strategies and approaches to health promotion found in the ENHPS and CSH models. The four elements of the CSH model – Instruction, Social Support, Social Services, Healthy Environments – are respectively reflected in the Convention. Article 24, 2(e), reflects the CSH strategy of Instruction as it obligates ratifying governments to provide children and parents with access to education about their health – specifically with regard to nutrition, hygiene, and environmental sanitation (promotional health issues). Article 27, 3, requires that ratifying states provide material assistance and support programs (reflecting Social Support and Social Services) to ensure children's rights to a standard of living conducive to their full physical, mental, spiritual, moral, and social development (holistic health goals). Finally, Article 24, 2(c) supports the creation of Healthy Environments for children and, in fact, obligates States Parties to take measures to ensure that environments allow children to achieve the highest attainable standard of health (United Nations 1989).

Likewise, many ENHPS principles guiding the practice of health promotion are also found in the Convention. The principles of equity, empowerment, and democracy in the learning process and environment are strongly supported throughout the Convention, most notably in Article 2 (Non-discrimination), Article 5 (Recognition of children's evolving capacities to exercise rights and freedoms), and Articles 12 through 15 (which assert children's rights to form opinions and to exercise freedom of expression, thought, conscience, religion, and association). The ENHPS view that curriculum should act as a stimulus for students' personal and professional development is directly reflected in sub-paragraphs (a) and (d) of Article 29, which, respectively, state that education shall be directed to "the development of the child's personality, talents and mental and physical abilities to their fullest potential" and "the preparation of the child for responsible life in a free society." Finally, the ENHPS model recognizes that the achievement of health requires measures at the physical, social, and community levels, and this view is supported throughout the Convention in references to the multiple determinants of children's health, well-being, and development (United Nations 1989).

The CSH and ENHPS can thus be seen as health promotion models that are in fact supported by international health and human rights organizations and by the consensus of a great number of countries. Recognition of the compatibility of the CSH and ENHPS models with the standards and approaches promoted by the WHO and the UN may serve to more broadly promote the use of these models as policy frameworks that can, and do, address the complex relationship between education and health.

In contrast to approaches whose orientation might be described as prescriptive or like a blueprint, the CSH and ENHPS models suggest viewing health promotion, from an educational perspective, as a "greenprint": that is, health promotion is "grown" from the inside out to reflect the local character, needs, and ambitions of the community it serves. For example, in Saskatchewan, educators are already talking about School PLUS, "a term coined by the Task Force on the Role of the School that describes a new conceptualization of schools" (Government of Saskatchewan 2004), as a way to broaden thinking about the delivery of health and community services (medical, psychological, social, police, adult learning) and the opportunities that schools offer as centres of learning for the entire community (Tymchak 2001). In Prince Edward Island, educators are in the process of coordinating health and social services, education, justice, and career advancement under the umbrella of the Active Healthy School Communities (AHSC) Program. This is truly a much more comprehensive understanding of health and education in which educational improvement and health promotion use community building to increase local capacity for change. We now discuss the application of these health promotion principles in schools.

IMPLEMENTING COMPREHENSIVE HEALTH PROMOTION POLICIES IN SCHOOLS: ISSUES AND CHALLENGES

School Structure and Size

Interestingly, as students progress through the school system from elementary to secondary school, their feelings of connectedness with the school diminish. Resnick, Harris, and Blum (1993) noted that adolescents who feel that their schools care about them and who feel that they belong at their school are less likely to engage in risky activities than are those who feel disconnected from their school.

These feelings are due largely to the overall structure of secondary schools (Lee and Loeb 2000). As students move from class to class, the changes in class composition and teacher with each subject make the creation of a stable social structure difficult. With 1,000 to 3,000 students attending a secondary school, and as many as 1,500 students attending an elementary school, a myriad of social dynamics can occur on any given day. Large enrolments present enormous problems in terms of safety, supervision, timetabling, resource access, and facility management. In small schools (of fewer than four hundred students), teachers tend to have a positive attitude about their responsibility for students' learning, and students learn more. In short, small schools are better not only for students but also for teachers. The critical concern for large schools is that students can become lost in the crowd. It is easy to be overlooked in the melee of day-to-day activities, unless school board administrators and teachers make concerted efforts to know students as people and to ensure that all students feel like they belong and contribute. Implementing health-promoting school programs in large schools can be a major challenge.

Activity and Nutrition

Nutritional deficiencies and poor health attributed to sedentary living habits in adolescents are among the causes of low school enrolment, high absenteeism, early dropout, and poor class performance. There are a number of reasons that account for young people's not eating breakfast before going to school. Among these reasons are lack of appropriate foods in the house, dieting regimens, family conflict, and lack of appetite due to late-night snacking. Students also may have to leave early to catch transport for school before they are ready to eat in the morning. Many elementary schools, in collaboration with community service groups, provide breakfast, lunch, and snack programs to ensure that younger students are properly nourished. Secondary schools rarely offer these programs to adolescents, who are in a period of rapid growth and need to eat several small portions a day to fuel their developmental needs.

Adolescents, especially young women, are not as active as they once were, nor are they as active as various guidelines recommend (Pate et al. 1995). Youths are increasingly sedentary, and only about 50% of Canadian youths participate in physical activity regularly and with sufficient intensity to generate a conditioning or health benefit (King, Boyce, and King 1999). Many youths spend a great deal of time watching television and playing video games, activities that may be correlated with the consumption of high-calorie junk foods that have little nutrient value.

School physical activity programs, both curricular and extra-curricular, offer students protection from cardiovascular disease, diabetes, osteoporosis, some cancers, hypertension, and obesity (US Department of Health and Human Services 1996). The school physical education program may be the only opportunity that *all* adolescents have to engage in a balanced, health-educative program. Quality physical education programs, presented by qualified and enthusiastic teachers, ensure that students are vigorously active in developmentally appropriate experiences that enable them to progressively develop the knowledge and skills associated with leading a healthy active life. Large schools, however, can present a major challenge in the implementation of good physical activity programs and/or nutritional programs (Lee and Loeb 2000).

The Content and Approach of Health Curricula

Health has been a mandated area of study in the overall school curriculum since the beginnings of school systems across Canada. The content for study, influenced by various health, social, civic, and political movements outside the school system, has responded in the past to the threat of infectious diseases as well as to the anti-alcohol concerns of the temperance movement. More recently, public concerns about reducing the incidence of teenage pregnancy, sexually transmitted diseases, and violence have influenced school health curricula. Very little attention is paid, however, to other critical issues, such as how poverty affects people's decisions about smoking or how issues of race and gender relate to opportunities for health. Issues such as homosexuality and abortion, sexual pleasure and desire are also conspicuously absent. Furthermore, examination of curriculum documents reveals very little reference to spiritual health in a non-denominational sense. The education system is just not yet ready to tackle these discussions in classrooms, despite the fact that students want to know more about these issues (McCall et al. 1999).

Smith and Peterat (2000) examined the underlying assumptions that have guided health education practices in schools over the last century. They categorized approaches to health education under the following headings: factual and transmission, factual and transactional, interpretive and transactional, critical and transformational. Underlying each of these approaches to health education are

Table 5.3
Key areas of study within new health education curriculum documents

NUTRITION	relating nutritious eating to healthy lifestyles, weight management, body image, cultural and ethnic diversity, strategies for dealing with social pressures about food choices, eating disorders, and disordered eating
SAFETY AND INJURY PREVENTION	recognizing actions that promote road, vehicle, playground, and home safety; violence prevention dealing with harassment and assault, gangs, bullying, conflict resolution; fire prevention, sun protection
PHYSICAL ACTIVITY DEVELOPMENT	building knowledge and skills for participation in a wide variety of fitness, sports, recreational pursuits; cooperation, goal setting, and fair play
HUMAN GROWTH AND DEVELOPMENT	understanding physical, social, and emotional maturation, human sexuality, healthy relationships, birth control, prevention of sexually transmitted diseases, and abstinence

fundamental assumptions and beliefs about the contributions schools make to society through health education programs, what content is worth knowing (and what is left out), and what it means to be an educated person. Study that entails transformational learning experiences, for example, requires students to engage in critical and analytic modes of thinking and discussion about health. Factual or "transmission" learning tends to require only mental absorption of details and information provided directly by the teacher or textbooks. Health promotion is usually critical and interpretive in nature. Health studied from a multidisciplinary perspective includes an understanding of the social, political, and economic factors that affect daily living (e.g., how gendered and cultural views of the world influence decisions for health, how religion and ritual relate to perceptions of health, and the relationship between the causes of illness and the ability to engage in health promotion practices).

Other current health promotion curricula in schools focus on the development of life skills – problem solving, decision making, conflict management, and coping skills as well as self-esteem training – to empower students to think critically and analytically in relation to social and health issues. Exemplary programs extend beyond the individual to consider surrounding influences: family, culture, media, and living standards. Table 5.3 presents key areas of study within new health education curriculum documents. Educational psychologists have urged educators to take into account, when providing instruction in these skills and issues, how students' thinking is formed in relation to their backgrounds, experiences, beliefs, and goals. Case studies, role-playing activities, reflective journal writing, and portfolios have sometimes replaced textbooks. Increasingly, students are widening the scope of their discussions about health to include determinants of health and well-being, such as peace, the economy, policy, and government.

There is no evidence to suggest, however, that these changes are happening pervasively. On a positive note, worldwide discussions have begun to form around the notion of health literacy, which has been defined by one American organization as "the capacity of individuals and groups to obtain, interpret, and understand basic health information and services and the competence to use such information and services in ways that enhance health" (Joint Committee on National Health Education Standards 1995, 5). Four dimensions identified as essential to health literacy are: critical thinking, effective communication, self-directed learning, and responsible citizenry. These four dimensions constitute not only education for health but also education that prepares students to think carefully, resourcefully, and responsibly. Recent discussions of literacy have extended the concept to put greater emphasis on empowerment and action for change. Nutbeam (2000) has proposed a three-level hierarchy in health literacy: basic/functional literacy, communicative/interactive literacy, and critical literacy. He argues that achieving the level of critical literacy encourages greater autonomy and personal empowerment, which is also an important goal for education.

Health education is usually taught as part of the physical education, family studies, or guidance program. It may also be offered in other areas of academic study through thematic studies (e.g., friendship, multiculturalism) or as interdisciplinary studies (e.g., HIV/AIDS with history, economics, biology, sociology, health). Teachers, however, have very little formal training for teaching health education (Anderson and Massey 1998). Pre-service and in-service training for health tends to be a low priority area of professional development.

Advancements in instruction and materials for teaching health education have been generated by Health Canada, professional associations in education and public health, non-government organizations such as the Centre for Addiction and Mental Health and the Heart and Stroke Foundation, and community health professionals.

Due to protests by some religious or ethnic communities, certain study topics are either omitted or presented using outdated teacher-centred methods, such as lectures, videos, and whole class discussions (McCall et al. 1999). Students enrolled in sexual health education programs complain that teachers focus too much on anatomy, pregnancy, and condom use, while leaving out topics such as relationships, abuse and sexual assault, STD prevention, birth control methods and abortion, sexual orientation and "coming out," affection, attraction, love, sex, and alcohol use. Students have also called for more active learning/teaching methods that enable them to explore ideas and issues personally, interpersonally, and across communities.

Stakeholder Participation in Policy and Program Development

Hargreaves (1994) suggests that having a coherent and validated set of policy principles, as illustrated in the ENHPS and CSH, does not necessarily produce a viable program on its own: "[p]olicy is best secured, not through the sole medium of written administrative texts, but through communities of people within and across schools who create policies, talk about them, process them, inquire into them, and reformulate them, bearing in mind the circumstances and children they know best" (5).

Policy formation should be born out of a process that involves clarifying and declaring values, purposes, and visions. School policies should evolve as understandings about the teaching/learning process continue to change, as we learn and appreciate new ideas about how best to teach, as we learn more about how student backgrounds and experiences interact with classroom experiences, and as technological advances give us greater access to ways in which to communicate.

The struggle lies in trying to move from a position in which stakeholders are merely implementers or tools of other people's policies to a position in which they realize policies, making them their own. Health promotion principles envisioned in ENHPS, such as democracy, equity, empowerment, collaboration, and partnership, encourage stakeholder participation in formulating policies appropriate to their needs. The ENHPS model enables educators to discuss, revise, validate, expand, authenticate, and inquire about the health and educational vitality of their work in schools.

Strong, positive, collaborative school cultures also have powerful and positive effects on the academic and behavioural functioning of young people (De Wit et al. 2000). Effective schools create cultures that: share visions and goals with stakeholders, are devoted to the creation of learning environments for everyone, set high expectations that all work hard to reach; value good teaching, and attend to the rights and responsibilities of students' as leaders and partners. Teachers and students succeed in school cultures that focus on participation and involvement, meaning and moral purpose, leadership and advocacy (Sammons, Hillman, and Mortimore 1995).

The Role of School Management

School principals play a pivotal role in the way schools operate. Those who are committed to health promotion ensure the health curriculum is taught, ensure teachers are prepared to teach the content as it is prescribed, allocate the resources – time, materials, professional development – needed to support and enrich program delivery, and assess student achievement related to health expectations. In many instances, the health education curriculum is set aside because of the overwhelming emphasis on academic achievement. Unless policy at the board level is directed at monitoring curriculum delivery and measuring results, much of what needs to be taught in health education will remain a low priority. Further, if health is to have reach beyond the classroom, the entire school must become involved. Each school must be encouraged to create its own policies that articulate the values of health promotion, that reflect how the entire school can promote health, that involve students and community partners, and that set its own goals for health and school improvement. Each school's "greenprint" for action should reflect a collaborative effort on the part of teachers, pupils, community partners, and parents to create and mobilize school policies that integrate goals for health and education.

The Role of Teachers

Teachers can enjoy a special relationship with students that enhances the students' chances for success. This relationship is strengthened by ensuring that teachers are knowledgeable, skilled, and well-resourced. Investments in teacher development related to health education offer untold dividends for both students and teachers. Research has demonstrated that, with support, teachers can:

- recognize students as sources of knowledge, not simply as consumers;
- treat all students with respect;
- empower students to become lifelong learners by teaching them not only content but strategies for interacting with concepts and ideas, how to communicate ideas and information based on their personal knowledge and experiences, and how to organize information and ideas (Wilkins and Tryfos 2000);
- set and maintain high expectations for themselves and students;
- work creatively and collaboratively with students, colleagues, parents, and professional communities to attain these high expectations; and
- relate research (their own and others') to practice, with the aim of improving their teaching (Darling-Hammond 1995; 1998).

What is important about policy development in this process is that teachers, as the key professionals in education, assume ownership and authority over school improvements. Policy decisions created at the local level, where teachers have to actualize them, are more likely to be carried out.

Student Involvement

Increasingly, students are activists for social change, health, and school improvement. By creating opportunities for youths to put their skills into action, they become recognized as valued and effective community members. Student involvement strengthens the overall capacity of the school and surrounding community for ongoing and sustained educational improvement.

Ontario Students Against Impaired Driving (www.osaid.org) is one example of many student-led efforts to alert fellow youths to the dangers of driving while impaired. Students also organize outreach programs that help the homeless, help each other through peer support study and counselling programs, and raise funds for research and community improvement projects. Many schools provide student-led training for CPR and host health awareness seminars related to the prevention of diabetes, cancer, heart disease, and HIV/AIDS. Youth-driven social action is a way for young people to participate as agents of change, health activists, and contributing members of their society.

Role of the Local Health and Service Sectors

Local health sectors and schools have worked together for decades towards improving and sustaining the health of adolescents. The most common roles played by local health sectors in schools have been as providers of:

- screening and treatment services;
- consultancy and advocacy for school personnel, students, and parents on health issues and approaches to school-based health promotion;
- policy development concerning specific issues such as allergies or HIV/AIDS; and
- technical support for education and training of teachers to improve their health knowledge and skills and curriculum resource materials.

The school nurse has always been a welcome partner in health education, but due to resource cutbacks in the Canadian health sector, fewer nurses are available and their job descriptions no longer provide for as much interaction with students in the classroom, parents, or teachers.

Police and fire departments, the criminal justice system, and citizenry and social service departments have also worked with educators to develop and implement a wide range of prevention policies and programs related to smoking, violence, suicide, substance abuse, and pollution. In some instances, there may be too many interested but uncoordinated groups developing materials. For example, there are currently over one hundred different organizations across Canada that have developed smoking prevention and cessation resource materials. If these materials are to be effective, they must be aligned with overall educational mandates and the existing characteristics of schools, teaching methods, and school cultures.

RECOMMENDATIONS FOR PROVINCIAL MINISTRIES, SCHOOL BOARDS, AND SCHOOLS

The following recommendations for the development of comprehensive school health promotion policy are related to three jurisdictions; namely, the province, the school board, and the school.

At the provincial ministry level, policy-makers should:

(a) facilitate a process that enables school districts, schools, teachers, and administrators to craft an educational version of health promotion that reflects their needs, strengths, and goals;

(b) foster collaborative research activities that universities, schools, and teachers design together (e.g., in Australia, as an incentive, the government distributes grants to help schools operationalize research plans for their school);

(c) intensify the contribution that university faculties of education make to teacher preparation for health education (there are a number of faculties of education across Canada that do not include health education as part of their initial teacher preparation programs; few faculties have tenured faculty dedicated to curriculum and instruction for health education);

(d) build a relationship between federal health ministry and provincial education and health ministries (the federal government is reluctant to sponsor research or fund projects in schools because education is a provincial matter; little research is funded by either the provincial ministries of health or education that investigates effective methods of promoting or implementing Comprehensive School Health in schools);

(e) build capacity for ongoing improvement through data-gathering strategies that build understanding, engage participants in a process of valuation versus evaluation, and personalize and localize progress by gathering stories and first-hand accounts in addition to statistical data; and

(f) enable school boards to organize course offerings, learning opportunities, timetables, and course loads in such a way that physical and health education programs and programs for the arts are not crowded out by "core" subjects (ministries of education should resource school boards so that creative alternatives to subject matter study beyond the regular school day are affordable, efficient, and effective for all schools).

At the school board level, authorities should:

(a) promote development of health promotion/school improvement plans;

(b) activate meaningful partnerships with parents, youth organizations, community health professionals, non-government organizations, professional associations, and municipal agencies (housing, employment services, and legal and psychological counselling);

(c) provide health-promoting physical environments for both working and learning, through school buildings, playgrounds, and food services;

(d) ensure that students and staff can learn and work in a safe school, free from discrimination, harassment, and violence;

(e) ensure that students can participate in a quality health education program despite curriculum overload (all students should graduate knowing how to manage health decisions);

(f) ensure that students can participate in a quality physical education program despite curriculum overload (by restructuring user fees and supporting innovative programming, timetabling, and facility usage); and

(g) coordinate access to community health, social, and protection services for families of school-aged children.

At the school level, authorities should:

(a) expose students to the United Nations Convention on the Rights of the Child and its implications for their lives;

(b) create opportunities to find out what students have to say and put mechanisms in place to explore how students feel about themselves, their relationships with peers at school, their sense of belonging in school, and their relationships with teachers (students' ideas, beliefs, and concerns can be expressed through printed materials, multimedia exhibitions, systematic inquiry, and action research methods);

(c) respect and promote student voices; enable students to play an important role in school governance, student services, curriculum reform, assessment and evaluation practices, and community outreach; collect stories, pictures, cartoons, and anecdotal information and display these using murals, websites, and school newsletters; collect information not only from students but also from teachers and administrators; and ask the questions:

   (i) What makes life good for you and the people you care about at school?

    (ii) What makes life not so good for you and those you care about at school?

    (iii) What would make things better at school?

(d) ensure that students learn under the supervision and direction of qualified, enthusiastic teachers;

(e) ensure that all students can participate in health-promoting extracurricular activities (e.g., drama, athletics, music, outdoor adventure, citizenship clubs) as part of an inclusive school; and

(f) invite a panel of experts, such as students, teachers, psychologists, and social workers, to participate in an open dialogue about key school issues (e.g., violence), and note that such discussion and dialogue should influence public and political discourses occurring in the legislative assemblies and in the media.

CONCLUSIONS

This chapter has presented a number of key strategic improvements to schools that can strengthen this basic health determinant and result in improved health for adolescents. These strategies include:

- maximizing opportunities present in the physical environment to contribute to the health of those involved with the school;
- maximizing the potential of the school culture to contribute to a supportive learning environment in which healthy relationships and the emotional well-being of students are valued and strengthened;
- promoting active student participation in formal curriculum and decision making processes of the school;
- developing a range of lifelong health-related skills and knowledge;
- enhancing equality in education and health by realizing the health competencies of all members of the school community;
- providing a positive and supportive working environment for those who work in schools;
- enabling the school and the local community to collaborate in health initiatives to benefit students, their families, and community members; and
- strengthening families by encouraging their involvement in the management of the school and their participation in the development of health skills and knowledge in their children.

It is common for governments to focus educational policy on individual performance, such as curriculum expectations that outline what students should know and be able to do. Yet policy rarely focuses on the school conditions that affect this performance. Standardized tests that focus on very narrow measures of achievement fail to represent what schools do and what society values about education. Other education policy has been aimed at cutting costs through school closures and increasing administrative efficiency. Yet such policy rarely focuses on fostering adventurous and innovative ways for schools to operate and for teachers to teach. Changing the behaviour of the organization, reinvigorating school environments, supporting the way teachers work and learn, and observing the ways that schools and communities interact are strategies that remain conspicuously absent from the policy-making process. Refocusing schools to reflect the principles of health-promoting strategic models like the CSH or ENHPS, for example, requires bold and aggressive steps initiated at multiple levels of action: provincial governments, school boards, administrators, and teachers. All of these stakeholders must cooperate to ensure strengthening of the school's capacity in governance, curriculum design, and instructional delivery and in creating a healthy learning environment.

REFERENCES

Allensworth, D. 1993. Health education: State of the art. *Journal of School Health* 63(1):14–20.
Anderson, A. 1999. Using health education to develop literacy. *Research for Educational Reform* 4(1):21–33.
– 2000. Teaching health for understanding. *Avante* 6(2):105–114.
Anderson, A., I. Kalnins, D. McCall, and D. Raphael. 1999. *Partners for Health: Schools, Communities, and Young People Working Together.* Ottawa: Health Canada.
Anderson, A., and D. Massey. 1998. Developing health education learning outcomes for beginning teachers (non-specialist) using the Delphi technique. *Avante* 4(2):39–48.
Anderson, A., and N. Piran. 2001. Health-promoting schools: Guiding principles of an international movement. *Orbit* 31(4):4–9.

Canadian Association for School Health (CASH). 1991. *Comprehensive School Health: A Framework for Cooperative Action. A National Consensus Statement.* White Rock, BC: CASH.

Connop, H., and A.J.C. King. 1999. *Young Women at Risk.* Toronto: University of Toronto Press.

Darling-Hammond, L. 1995. Policy for restructuring. In *The Work of Restructuring Schools,* ed. A. Lieberman, 157–75. New York: Teachers College Press.

– 1998. Teacher learning that supports student learning. *Educational Leadership* 55(5):6–11.

De Wit, D., D. Offord, B. Rye, M. Shain, and R. Wright. 2000. The effect of school culture on adolescent behavioural problems: Self-esteem, attachment to learning, and peer approval of deviance as mediating mechanisms. *Canadian Journal of School Psychology* 16(1):15–38.

Dryfoos, J. 1990. *Adolescents at Risk: Prevalence and Prevention.* New York: Oxford University Press.

Glazier, R.H., E.M. Badley, J.E. Gilbert, and L. Rothman. 2000. The nature of increased hospital use in poor neighbourhoods: Findings from a Canadian inner city. *Canadian Journal of Public Health* 91:268–273.

Government of Saskatchewan. 2004. *School PLUS: Giving Saskatchewan Students What They Need to Succeed.* http://www.schoolplus.gov.sk.ca/pe/main/about. Retrieved 19 July 2006.

Hargreaves, A. 1994. The changing world of teaching in the 1990s. *Orbit* 25(4):2–5.

Jessor, R. 1993. Successful adolescent development among youth in high-risk settings. *American Psychologist* 48:117–126.

Joint Committee on National Health Education Standards. 1995. *Achieving Health Literacy: An Investment in the Future.* Atlanta: American Cancer Society.

King, A.J., W.F. Boyce, and M.A. King. 1999. *Trends in the Health of Canadian Youth.* Cat. no. H39498/1999E. Ottawa: Health Canada.

Kolbe, L. 1985. Why school health promotion? An empirical point of view. *Health Education* 16:20–4.

– 1986. Increasing the impact of school health promotion perspectives: Emerging research perspectives. *Health Education* 17:47–52.

Lavin, A.T., G.R. Shapiro, and K.S. Weill. 1992. Creating an agenda for school-based health promotion: A review of 25 selected reports. *Journal of School Health* 62:212–29.

Lee, V., and S. Loeb. 2000. School size in Chicago elementary schools: Effects on teachers' attitudes and student achievement. *American Educational Research Journal* 37(1):3–32.

Marx, E., S. Wooley, and D. Northrop, eds. 1998. *Health Is Academic: A Guide to Coordinated School Health Programs*. New York: Teachers College Press.

McCall, D. 1999. Comprehensive school health: Help for teachers from the community. *Canadian Association for Health, Physical Education, Recreation, and Dance* 65(1):4–9.

McCall, D., R. Beasley, M. Doherty-Poirier, C. Lovato, D. MacKinnon, J. Otis, and M. Shannon. 1999. *Schools, Public Health, Sexuality and HIV: A Status Report*. Toronto: Councils of Ministers of Education (Canada).

National Health and Medical Research Council (NHMRC) Health Advancement Standing Committee. 1996. *Effective School Health Promotion: Towards Health Promoting Schools* [rescinded 2005]. N.p.: NHMRC (Australia).

Nutbeam, D. 2000. Health literacy as a public health goal: A challenge for contemporary health education and communication strategies into the 21st century. *Health Promotion International* 15:259–68.

– 2002. Finding common ground in health and education: The Healthy Schools Programme. In *Education and Health in Partnership*, 41–44. Conference Report. Woerden: NIGZ (Netherlands Institute for Health Promotion and Disease Prevention).

O'Loughlin, J.L., Paradis, G., K. Gray-Donald, and L. Renauld. 1999. The impact of a community-based heart disease prevention program in a low-income, inner-city neighbourhood. *American Journal of Public Health* 89:1819–26.

Pate, R.R., M. Pratt, S.N. Blair, W.L. Haskell, C.A. Macera, C. Bouchard, D. Buchner, W. Ettinger, G.W. Heath, A.C. King, A. Kriska, A.S. Leon, B.H. Marcus, J. Morris, R.S. Paffenberger, K. Patrick, M.L. Pollack, J.M. Rippe, J. Sallis, and J.H. Wilmore. 1995. Physical activity and public health: A recommendation from the Centers for Disease Control and Prevention and the American College of Sports Medicine. *Journal of the American Medical Association* 273(5):402–7.

Resnick, M.D., L.J. Harris, and R.W. Blum. 1993. The impact of caring and connectedness on adolescent health and well-being. *Journal of Paediatrics and Child Health* 29(Suppl 1):S3–9.

Rudd, R.E., and D.C. Walsh. 1993. Schools as healthful environments: Prerequisites to comprehensive school health. *Preventive Medicine* 22:499–506.

Rutter, M. 1979. *Fifteen Thousand Hours: Secondary Schools and Their Effects on Children*. Cambridge, MA: Harvard University Press.

Sammons, P., J. Hillman, and P. Mortimore. 1995. *Characteristics of Effective Schools: A Review of School Effectiveness Research*. London, UK: Office for Standards in Education (Ofsted).

Smith, W.J., and C. Lusthaus. 1994. Equal education opportunity for students with disabilities in Canada: The right to free and appropriate education. *Exceptionality Education Canada* 4:37–73.

Smith, G., and L. Peterat. 2000. Reading between the lines: Examining assumptions in health education. In *Weaving Connections: Educating for Peace, Social and Environmental Justice*, ed. Tara Goldstein and David Selby, 242–67. Toronto: Sumach Press.

St Leger, L. 2001. Schools, health literacy and public health: Possibilities and challenges. *Health Promotion International* 16(2):197–205.

St Leger, L., and D. Nutbeam. 2000. A model for mapping linkages between health and education agencies to improve school health. *Journal of School Health* 70:45–50.

Stephens, T., and D. Fowler Graham, eds. 1993. *Canada's Health Promotion Survey 1990: Technical Report*. Cat. no. H39–263/2–1990E. Ottawa: Minister of Supply and Services Canada.

ten Dam, G. 2002. Effectiveness of linking education with the promotion of health in schools. In *Education and Health in Partnership*, 17–22. Conference Report. Woerden: NIGZ (Netherlands Institute for Health Promotion and Disease Prevention).

Tymchak, M. 2001. *School PLUS: A Vision for Children and Youth*. Task Force and Public Dialogue on the Role of the School. Final Report to the Minister of Education. Regina: Government of Saskatchewan.

United Nations. 1989. *Convention on the Rights of the Child*. Geneva: United Nations.

United States Department of Health and Human Services. 1996. *Physical Activity and Health: A Report of the Surgeon General*. Atlanta, GA: US Department of Health and Human Services, Centers for Disease Control and Prevention, National Center for Chronic Disease Prevention and Health Promotion.

Valpy, M. 1993. Drafting the village to help the schools. *Globe and Mail*, February.

Wilkins, C., and B. Tryfos. 2000. *Reaching Higher: Supporting Student Achievement in Literacy*. Mississauga, Ontario: Peel District School Board.

World Health Organization (WHO). 1986. *Ottawa Charter for Health Promotion*. First International Conference on Health Promotion, Ottawa, 21 November. WHO/HPR/HEP/95.1. Geneva: WHO. http://www.who.int/hpr/NPH/docs/ottawa_charter_hp.pdf). Retrieved 17 July 2006.

– 1995. *Promoting Health through Schools*. Report of a WHO Expert Committee on Comprehensive School Health Education and Promotion. Geneva: WHO. http://dosei.who.int/uhtbin/cgisirsi/pCcti9u2bX/306910020/9. Retrieved 17 July 2006.

6

The Health and Well-being of Aboriginal Youths in Canada

HARRIET MacMILLAN, CORNELIA WIEMAN,
ELLEN JAMIESON, ANGUS MacMILLAN,
AND CHRISTINE WALSH

INTRODUCTION

All Aboriginal cultures teach that children are special gifts lent by the
spirit world; if they are not loved and cherished, they may flee back to
the realm from which they came.

Fournier and Crey 1997, 81

Many reports about Canadian Aboriginal youth emphasize the
importance of understanding the health status and needs of this
unique and diverse group (Stout and Kipling 1999; Kidder et al.
2000), yet there is a paucity of rigorous data available (MacMillan,
MacMillan, et al. 1996; Offord et al. 1989). Much of the published
literature is based on studies involving United States Native groups
(Offord et al. 1989). As highlighted by Waldram, Herring, and
Young (1995), while many large national health surveys have been
conducted in Canada over the past thirty years, most have excluded
persons living on-reserve. Although the national Aboriginal Peoples
Survey (APS) was conducted by Statistics Canada in 1991, the study
was not conducted in collaboration with First Nations and/or Inuit
representatives (Statistics Canada 1991, 1992, 1993a, 1993b).
Furthermore, the APS concentrated only on persons 15 years of age
and older.

Collaborative research helps to ensure that issues are relevant to
Aboriginal people (Beiser 1981) and may increase participation levels
(Federal, Provincial, and Territorial Advisory Committee on Population

Health 1999). The recent First Nations and Inuit Regional Health Survey (FNIRHS) (First Nations and Inuit Regional Health Survey National Steering Committee 1999) was initiated to compensate for the exclusion of Aboriginal people living on reserves from the sampling frame of previous Canadian longitudinal surveys, including the National Longitudinal Survey of Children and Youth (NLSCY) (HRDC and Statistics Canada 1996). The FNIRHS represents an important step towards examining the health status of Aboriginal people generally; however, the core section on child (age newborn to 11 years) and youth (age 12 to 17 years) health was limited to ten questions. Only Manitoba, Nova Scotia, and Ontario included an additional section that focused in more depth on the health status of youth.

Other chapters in this book refer to the Health Behaviour in School-aged Children (HBSC) survey, which provides no information about the health issues of Aboriginal youth (King, Boyce, and King 1999), although a question has been added in the most recent 2002 HBSC questionnaire to capture information about ethnicity. The need to address the lack of rigorous information about the health of Aboriginal youth is compounded by the fact that what data are available suggest that Aboriginal youths are among the most disadvantaged of all Canadians (Hanvey 1994). Even less is known about the strengths of Aboriginal youth and the factors associated with resiliency, which has been measured infrequently. These gaps in knowledge already identify a key issue that has important policy implications – the urgent need for comprehensive, population-based information about the physical, social, and emotional health of Aboriginal youths.

The sections that follow summarize what is known from the available peer-reviewed literature as well as selected reports, including the Final Reports of the Nova Scotia First Nations Regional Health Survey (NSFNRHS) (Mi'kmaq Health Research Group 1999), the Ontario First Nations Regional Health Survey (OFNRHS) (MacMillan, Walsh, Faries, et al. 1998), and the First Nations and Inuit Regional Health Survey (FNIRHS) (First Nations and Inuit Regional Health Survey National Steering Committee 1999). A comprehensive literature review was conducted using MEDLINE, PsycINFO, and Sociofile to November 2001. Selected US studies were included for those areas where comparable Canadian data were not available or where the sample was sufficiently broad-based that the findings might be relevant to Canadian Aboriginal youth. The National Aboriginal Health

Organization (NAHO) provided the authors with recent unpublished reports that included a focus on Aboriginal youth. Comparisons with non-Aboriginal data have been made where Canadian information was relevant (community-based studies, analogous age groups, comparable measures) and available: no new analyses of data (e.g., later cycles of the NLSCY) were undertaken.

In this chapter, the term "Aboriginal" is used to refer to people whose ancestors were indigenous to Canada. Within Canada, there are three broad categories of Aboriginal groups: First Nations, Inuit, and Métis (Webster 2000). The term "Indian" is sometimes still used to refer to First Nations persons, even though many Aboriginal people find it to be offensive when applied to Native Canadians. Hence this term is used exclusively when required to accurately describe information from an original source. The designation "Registered" or "Status" indicates an Aboriginal person who is registered under the Indian Act of Canada. Status Native bands are referred to as First Nations. A band is both a political organization and a cultural group (Kidder et al. 2000). Some research reported in this chapter refers only to specific groups of Aboriginal people – for example, First Nations persons living on-reserve – and is not intended to be generalized to all Aboriginals in Canada.

The first section provides a historical perspective on the lives of Canadian Aboriginal youths. To understand the current health issues of these youths, it is essential to review the historical, socio-economic, cultural, and political factors that have "woven a picture of significant health status inequities for Aboriginal peoples in Canada" (Postl et al. 1994, 41). This is followed by a summary of socio-demographic data regarding Canadian Aboriginal youths. The sections on determinants of health and specific aspects of health highlight those areas where information is available and identify important concepts about which little is known. The final section summarizes future directions and outlines some draft recommendations arising from the information reviewed; however, the authors recognize that definitive recommendations arising from this material must be determined by Aboriginal people themselves.

HISTORICAL PERSPECTIVE

Just as there are varied and diverse Aboriginal communities and nations within this country, so there is a heterogeneity in the experiences of Aboriginal youths. Given this diversity, it is sometimes difficult to clearly identify consistent themes or issues of concern regarding youths for fear of making over-generalizations. Nevertheless, despite the limitations of the literature, there are several common themes that do emerge in the contemporary experiences of Aboriginal youths. These themes can be better understood when put into a historical perspective. Around the time of contact with Europeans, estimates of the Aboriginal population vary from 500,000 to over 2 million (Dickason 1997). While the decline in Aboriginal numbers postcontact has been well described, for the past several decades, beginning in the 1950s and 1960s, the total number of individuals of Aboriginal ancestry in Canada has begun to increase in an exponential fashion, making it the fastest-growing segment of the Canadian population (Statistics Canada 1996). Currently, Aboriginal people account for approximately 2.8% of Canada's total population. It is expected that, by 2016, over 1.1 million people will be of Aboriginal ancestry (Statistics Canada 1996). Even these numbers are an underestimate, given the limitations of the census process, including exclusion or incomplete enumeration of some Aboriginal communities as well as the refusal of some Aboriginal individuals to self-identify (Kidder et al. 2000).

As discussed below, the Aboriginal population is heavily skewed towards the younger age groups. Children and youth (birth to nineteen years) represent 44% of the Aboriginal population but only 28% of the national population (Statistics Canada 1996). The increasing numbers of Aboriginal youths mean that their issues of concern will only rise to greater significance with the passage of time. As Postl (1997) writes, while a population suffers under both chronic health and social illnesses, the children are the most vulnerable and they grow first into adolescents then into adults. When all of their suffering and privations are coupled with decreased educational opportunities, low self-esteem, and poverty, the result is a cohort of young people who carry an "especially terrible burden" (1655).

Any examination of the contemporary realities of youths must take into consideration their families of origin, their parenting, and developmental experiences. For many Aboriginal youths, their development is tempered by the intergenerational impact of socially oppressive and culturally destructive historical events, such as the residential school system and the Sixties Scoop. Residential schools for Aboriginal youth in Canada officially operated between 1892 and 1969, and reached a peak of eighty-eight schools operating in the 1930s. The last residential school closed in British Columbia in 1983. It is estimated that up to one-third of all Aboriginal children attended residential schools between the mid-1800s through the 1970s (Fournier and Crey 1997; Assembly of First Nations 1998). The racism, cultural persecution, and various abuses (physical, emotional, sexual) experienced by many of the children and youths who attended residential schools have been well described. Likewise, the Sixties Scoop refers to the accelerated removal of children from their birth families by child welfare/protection agencies that began during the 1960s. It is estimated that, in the 1970s, one out of every four Status Indian children was either temporarily or permanently separated from their families. Many of these children suffered losses and abuses similar to those suffered by children who attended residential schools (Fournier and Crey 1997). Both the residential school experience and the Sixties Scoop are legislatively authorized examples of attempts by the Government of Canada to assimilate Aboriginal peoples; and, from the perspective of Aboriginal youth, successive generations of families have been negatively affected. Kirmayer, Brass, and Tait (2000) provide further details about the social origins of distress among First Nations people, including youth, and outline some of the factors that contribute to the continuing political marginalization of Aboriginal peoples.

In traditional settings, Aboriginal peoples respected the circularity of life, and both the young and the elderly were especially valued. There were special ceremonies, such as the Vision Quest, for Aboriginal adolescents on the cusp of young adulthood (Johnston 1982). Among other losses, deterioration of the traditional ways of parenting, fostering of cultural identity, and maintenance of cultural continuity, including maintenance of language and ceremonies, have resulted in the social and health consequences involving youth that are of present concern. The disparity between traditional culture and modern mainstream society is a real and ongoing challenge for today's Aboriginal youths.

The United Nations Convention on the Rights of the Child (UNCRC) addresses Aboriginal and indigenous children's rights. Article 30 (Children of minorities or indigenous peoples) notes that culture, language, and religion are key issues that are relevant to the well-being of youth. Other well-known determinants of Aboriginal youth health, however, such as social discrimination and economic status, are not mentioned directly. On the topic of culture, Chandler and Lalonde (1998) assert that the mechanism through which inadequate cultural expression affects youth health is lack of cultural continuity. This contributes to problems in self-continuity that can lead to suicide.

DETERMINANTS OF HEALTH

In order to understand their health issues, it is essential to have some knowledge about the conditions in which Aboriginal youths live. Much of this information is not specific to youths but must be extrapolated from data regarding Aboriginal people of all ages.

Based on 1996 Census figures, the population identifying themselves as Aboriginal is younger than the total Canadian population (Kidder et al. 2000). Within the total 1996 Aboriginal population (N = 799,010), 20% were between the ages of 10 and 19, while the comparable rate for the Canadian population (N = 28,528,125) was 14%. Aboriginal people are not distributed evenly across Canada: 81% are concentrated in Ontario, Manitoba, Saskatchewan, Alberta, and British Columbia. Only a small number live in the Yukon and Territorial regions, yet they constitute a substantial proportion of these regional populations; for example, within Nunavut, Canada's most recent northern territory, 87% of the population is Inuit (Kidder et al. 2000).

Economic Environment

According to the 1991 Aboriginal Peoples Survey, a large-scale survey of persons who reported Aboriginal heritage and/or being registered under the Indian Act, the unemployment rate among those 15 years of age and older was almost 25%, whereas the comparable rate in Canada's total population was 10% (Statistics Canada 1993b). The unemployment rate for Aboriginal youths aged 15 to 24 in 1996 was 32%, compared to 17% for non-Aboriginal youths (Kidder et al. 2000). As highlighted in the *Choosing Life* report of the Royal Commission on Aboriginal Peoples (RCAP), unemployment is considered a "serious contributing factor to both the mental and physical health problems of Canadians" (1995).

Although the level of educational achievement among Aboriginal people is still behind that of the total Canadian population, there have been some notable improvements in recent years. Data from the Department of Indian Affairs and Northern Development, cited in the Canadian Institute of Child Health report (Kidder et al. 2000), showed that the percentage of registered Indian on-reserve children and youth remaining in school for twelve consecutive years rose from 37% in 1987/1988 to 71% in 1996/1997. During this same period, the number of registered Indian and Inuit young people enrolled in postsecondary educational institutions rose from 14,000 to 27,000. This trend of increasing educational achievement is important, yet not widely recognized.

Physical Environment

Youths, especially those who follow a traditional lifestyle (Postl et al. 1994), are at risk for exposure to environmental toxins. Heavy metals, particularly mercury, lead, and organic chemicals, which include compounds such as polychlorinated biphenyl (PCB), pose considerable health threats to Aboriginal people across their lifespan (Dewailly et al. 1993). It is now apparent that a wide range of toxins continue to enter the food chain; while the specific effects of some contaminants are unknown, the theoretical hazards are concerning (Postl et al. 1994).

Aboriginal families experience problems associated with low socio-economic status, including poor housing, water management, and waste disposal. Based on the Canada Mortgage and Housing Corporation's standards of "housing need," a concept that takes into account crowding, need of repair, and affordability, 1996 Census data indicate that Aboriginal families with children are far more likely than are their non-Aboriginal counterparts to live in housing need (Kidder et al. 2000). Aboriginal families showed a threefold increase in likelihood of residing in homes with multiple problems related to housing. Although there have been few data available about the quality of drinking water, the final report of an inquiry into water quality in Walkerton, a rural community in Ontario, noted that eighty-three reserves across Canada, including twenty-two in Ontario, have water systems at high risk of contamination (Mackie 2002).

Regarding facilities available in the community, 42.2% of OFNRHS males and 50.2% of females reported that there were sports facilities available for boys in the community. A lesser proportion of both males (35.7%) and females (40.6%) indicated that there were sports facilities available for girls. Approximately one-third of males and females reported that there was a drop-in centre available for youth. Lower rates of male and female youths indicated the availability of a dance centre, music centre, or friendship centre.

A similar proportion of OFNRHS males (55.4%) and females (51.0%) reported the need for an arena, while 76.9% of males and 66.9% of females indicated the need for a swimming pool. More than 50% of both male and female youth respondents reported the need for a drop-in centre. An outdoor rink was described as needed by 56.9% of males and 39.4% of females. Playground equipment was reported as needed by 54% of male youths and 53.8% of female youths. Community halls and baseball diamonds were described as needed by approximately one-third of respondents.

HEALTH BEHAVIOURS

Nutrition

Moffatt (1995) has summarized information regarding nutritional deficiencies in Aboriginal people, which predominantly affect younger children rather than youths. These nutrients include iron, calcium, vitamin D, folate, vitamin A, and fluoride. He cautions that these data should not be generalized to all Aboriginal people and emphasizes that some communities have good nutrition. In the Aboriginal Peoples Survey, availability of food was reported as a problem by approximately 8% of respondents (Statistics Canada 1993b).

Although the OFNRHS did not focus on the nutrition of youths, several questions about nutritional health were asked of the youths in the Nova Scotia Survey of the Mi'kmaq population (Mi'kmaq Health Research Group 1999). While 87% of male and 94% of female youths indicated that healthy eating was either very or somewhat important to them, only 42% of male and 32% of female youths reported always eating breakfast. Furthermore, the self-report of youths about choice of lunch and snacks indicated a greater emphasis on less healthy foods. Comparable data from a Canada-wide household survey using twenty-four-hour recall interviews showed that adolescent (age 13 to 18) males, but not females, met Canada's Food Guide to Healthy Eating minimum recommended levels for all four food groups; for both genders, intake from the "other foods" group contributed over 25% of energy and fat (Starkey, Johnson-Down, and Gray-Donald 2001).

Obesity continues to be a major problem among Canada's Aboriginal youth. The results of the Nova Scotia and Ontario First Nations Regional Health Surveys indicate that a large proportion of youths weigh within the overweight and obese categories, based on self-report questionnaires. Parents in the FNIRHS, which included data from all regions except Alberta, indicated that 10.1% of youths aged 12 years and over were overweight (MacMillan, Walsh, Jamieson, et al. 1999). Obesity in adolescence is a predictor of adult obesity (Guo et al. 1994), which, in turn, increases the likelihood of such chronic diseases as type 2 diabetes mellitus and coronary heart disease (Hanley et al. 2000). Assessment of obesity in a sub-sample of First Nations youths aged 10 to 14 years of age living in Sandy Lake revealed that 23.5% of boys and 32.1% of girls were overweight (Hanley et al. 2000). The rates for those 15 to 19 years were 18.6% and 26.6%, respectively. Among youths 10 to 19 years of age, there was a strong inverse relationship between being overweight and both fitness level and fibre intake (in the previous twenty-four hours). The risk of being overweight rose with increased television viewing and consumption of junk food (in the previous three months). This study used anthropometric measurements rather than reliance on self-report information.

Substance Use

Substance abuse, including smoking and drug or alcohol abuse, among Aboriginal adolescents is a major issue of concern, although no national data are available about the extent of this problem. One Canadian survey compared rates of substance abuse between 1990 and 1993 among Native and white adolescents in a mid-western city (Gfellner and Hundleby 1995). With the exception of alcohol, a greater proportion of Native youths indicated use of substances, including marijuana, solvents, and hallucinogens, during each of the four years. Results from a Quebec study were similar (Lalinec-Michaud et al. 1991). In the NSFNRHS, 49% of female youths and 31% of male youths indicated that they had consumed alcohol in the past twelve months, while the rates for ever using alcohol among youth respondents to the OFNRHS were 63.3% for males and 68.8% for females. The alcohol use rates between Nova Scotia and Ontario First Nations youth are not comparable because the questions focused on different time periods of use. The Ontario Student Drug Use

Survey of about three thousand students in grades 7, 9, 11, and 13 showed rates of alcohol consumption in the past twelve months of 58.7%, 56.5%, 58.8%, 59.6%, and 56.7% in 1991, 1993, 1995, 1997, and 1999, respectively (Adlaf et al. 2000). Results were not tabulated by gender.

The OFNRHS youth self-report survey indicates that 63.2% of males and 62.4% of females smoked cigarettes in the last six months. Approximately two-thirds of Mi'kmaq youths reported using tobacco in non-traditional ways; 41% of male youths and 48% of female youths reported smoking cigarettes at the time of the survey. Previous surveys inquiring about the smoking patterns of Aboriginal youths from other Canadian regions indicate that smoking, and use of smokeless (chewing) tobacco, pose significant health problems (Pickering, Lavallee, and Hanley 1989; Millar 1990a, 1990b; Hoover, McDermott, and Hartsfield 1990; Lanier et al. 1990).

Among the OFNRHS youth, the rates for drug use were 54.2% for male youths and 48.1% for female youths. The rate of substance use based on youth self-report was uniformly higher than parent report of youth behaviours for all categories of substances. Among the NSFNRHS youth, 51% of males and 82% of females indicated that they had used drugs "at one time or another." The drugs used by the greatest proportion of youths were marijuana, hashish, pot, or grass, followed by some type of inhalant. The last drug has been identified as a major health problem in some regions, particularly in isolated Native communities (Muir 1988; Remington and Hoffman 1984).

In the United States, the National American Indian Adolescent Health Survey (Blum et al. 1992; Potthoff et al. 1998) collected more detailed information about frequency and intensity of substance abuse. Weekly or more frequent use of consumption of alcohol increased from 8.2% of Aboriginal youths in grade 7 to 14.1% among 12th graders. Other than alcohol, marijuana, peyote, and inhalants were the most common substances used. Interestingly, use of inhalants declined from 13.8% of 7th through 9th graders to 7% of high school students. An American study examining the sequence of substances used among a large sample of American Indian adolescents showed that alcohol was the most common initiating substance (Novins, Beals, and Mitchell 2001). Alcohol use was most often followed by marijuana, which typically preceded use of other drugs; however, marijuana and inhalants were also used as initiating substances.

SOCIAL ENVIRONMENT

Youth Identity

Any kid is trying to find him[-] or herself as an individual, but for Native youth there is the additional identity crisis of finding out who they are as a Native person.

Youth delegate (*Suicide Prevention Workshop* 1996, 6)

In *Choosing Life: Special Report on Suicide among Aboriginal Peoples* (RCAP 1995), the mechanisms by which Aboriginal identity for youth have been weakened include: (a) neglect or misrepresentation of Aboriginal history and culture in educational curriculum and the mass media; (b) racism; (c) loss of land, culture, language, and spirituality; (d) domination by mainstream European culture; and (e) individual experiences of maltreatment and discrimination. Aboriginal youths "describe both exclusion from the dominant society and alienation from the now idealized but once-real life on the land that is stereotypically associated with Aboriginality. The terrible emptiness of feeling strung between two cultures and psychologically at home in neither has been described" (RCAP 1995, 30). This erosion of identity has manifested itself in social difficulties, inequalities in the determinants of health, and various health problems expressed in physical, mental, emotional, and spiritual aspects. These issues exist for a significant proportion of Aboriginal youths as outlined in earlier sections of this chapter.

Given that essential elements of Aboriginal identity have been eroded for many years, there has been an increasing focus on determining approaches to strengthening the identity of Aboriginal youth. Work by Chandler and Lalonde (1998) in relation to suicide has focused on the importance of understanding how youth construct a sense of identity and the relationship with cultural continuity. While there is a general literature regarding factors associated with identity development in youth – for example, the presence of role models – those factors that are unique to strengthening identity in Aboriginal youth need to be understood. Chandler and Lalonde (1998) emphasize the need to examine the process of identity formation in First Nations youth, with a special focus on understanding how self-continuity may differ in persons of Native and non-Native culture.

It is important to involve Aboriginal youths directly in determining strategies to enhance youth identity, but in addition there is a need to highlight the role of young people more generally. As captured succinctly in *Choosing Life* (RCAP 1995), support for adolescents entails the recognition of their need to be taken seriously as having ideas of their own. It means finding ways to mobilize them to articulate and address their own (and by extension the community's) problems across a range of issues.

Traditional Culture

Regarding youth participation in Native cultural activities, over 60% of OFNRHS youths described speaking a Native language sometimes or often. Approximately 40% to 50% of youths described participating in traditional Native games, songs, dance, and stories. A majority of First Nations youths reported sometimes or often preparing traditional Native foods, participating in canoeing, or making traditional crafts. With respect to traditional dancing, almost 41% of males and approximately 36% of females reported that it was available in their community, while 40.2% of males and 36.1% of females indicated that drumming was available.

Results from the NSFNRHS were similar: 44% of youths indicated that they could speak Mi'kmaq "pretty well or better" and 59% reported being able to understand the language at least "pretty well or better" (Mi'kmaq Health Research Group 1999). A majority (62%) of Mi'kmaq youths reported participating in a traditional cultural event within the past twelve months. The most frequently attended event was the powwow, followed by smudging and sweetgrass ceremonies. In the FNIRHS, 67.6% of parents were very satisfied or satisfied with their youth's knowledge of Native culture (MacMillan, Walsh, Jamieson, et al. 1999).

Exposure to Violence

Although the majority of OFNRHS youths indicated that they never or rarely get hassled by other kids or older kids, 34.6% indicated that this happened sometimes or often. With regard to domestic violence, 17.4% indicated that they had seen or heard a parent hit an adult in their home sometimes or often; an additional 13%

indicated that this happened rarely. In response to a question about "an adult getting so mad or out of control you got hurt or you thought they were really going to hurt you badly," 68.8% indicated that this never happened, 15.4% reported that it happened rarely, and 10.6% reported that it happened sometimes or often. Almost 8% of youths reported that they were so bruised or hurt (as a result of the actions described in the previous question) that they had to see a doctor.

Regarding child maltreatment, OFNRHS respondents were asked about their experiences of physical and sexual abuse by an adult when they were "growing up." The definition of physical abuse included six categories, ranging from being pushed, grabbed, or shoved (often or sometimes) to being physically attacked (often, sometimes, or rarely). Exposure to being slapped or spanked, even if it occurred often, was not included in the definition of physical abuse. The definition of sexual abuse included four categories of unwanted experiences, ranging from being the victim of repeated indecent exposure by an adult to being sexually attacked. The definitions for both types of abuse included a broad range of exposures in terms of severity. Rates of childhood physical abuse self-reported by youths in the OFNRHS were high, with 36.2% of females and 33.1% of males reporting that they had been physically abused and 18.9% of females and 16.0% of males experiencing more severe physical abuse. Published data from the Ontario Mental Health Supplement (OHSUP), a 1990 community survey using the same self-report abuse questions, showed 19.6% of females and 23.8% of males aged 15 to 24 in the general population had experienced physical abuse; 8.5% of females and 8.3% of males had experienced severe physical abuse (MacMillan, Fleming, et al. 1997). In the OFNRHS, the father was cited most often as committing physical abuse (35.9%), followed by the mother (32.4%). Although persons outside the home were frequently reported as committing the physical abuse (stranger 20.5% and some other known person 15.3%), siblings were also endorsed as frequently committing physical abuse, with frequencies of 19.6% for older sisters and 15.4% for older brothers.

Reported rates for sexual abuse were also very high, with 28.4% of OFNRHS female youths and 14.0% of male youths reporting childhood sexual abuse. Furthermore, 27.8% of females and 7.0% of males reported severe sexual abuse. Comparable figures for the OHSUP general population group aged 15 to 24 were 9.3% for females and 2.2% for males for sexual abuse and 8.8% and 1.9% for severe sexual abuse for females and males, respectively (MacMillan, Fleming, et al. 1997). OFNRHS respondents reported that the majority of sexual abuse was committed by persons outside of the family; 63.5% of sexual abuse was committed by some other known person and 41.5% by a stranger. Although reports about Aboriginal youth often refer to the high rates of exposure to mal-treatment, to our knowledge, these are some of the few community-based data available about this major public health problem among Native young people.

HEALTH STATUS

In some areas regarding Aboriginal youth health, there is emerging evidence-based literature. For example, knowledge about the distribu-tion and determinants of suicide among Aboriginal youth is increas-ingly available (Kirmayer, Boothroyd, et al. 1999). Information about important general health-related issues, however, such as peer relation-ships, family relationships, and sexual identity (e.g., "two-spirited" youths whose gender is neither exclusively male nor exclusively female but, instead, contains both spirits) is almost non-existent. Furthermore, data regarding a wide range of conditions such as fetal alcohol syn-drome/fetal alcohol effects (Burd and Moffatt 1994; Bray and Anderson 1989), HIV/AIDS (Metler, Conway, and Stehr-Green 1991), and anti-social behaviour (e.g., involvement with gangs) are still extremely lacking. Different Aboriginal groups may have varying health issues; for example, rates of type 2 diabetes mellitus in adults vary signifi-cantly among groups (Inuit rates are generally lower than First Nations rates) and within groups (Young, Reading, et al. 2000).

The following sections summarize what is known about the major categories of Aboriginal youth health status: physical, emotional, and social. Although presented as separate sections, the fact that important overlaps exist across these categories is now well recog-nized in the general health literature. Much of the material that fol-lows focuses on health conditions or problems. Where possible, however, information about good health and improvement in func-tioning is highlighted. Indeed, progress has been made during the past thirty years in many areas of Aboriginal health, including that of youth (Ng 1996). These recent improvements notwithstanding, Aboriginal people in Canada still face a disproportionate number of serious health problems. For example, among youths 15 to 24 years of age, disability that may be linked with limitations in either physical or emotional health (or both) lasting at least six months was reported by 21.7% of Aboriginal youths compared to 7.0% of the total Canadian population (Ng 1996). Fortunately, the majority of disabilities were in the slight category (rather than moderate or severe), and only 6% of Aboriginal youths 15 to 24 years of age indicated having unmet needs requiring help with daily activities.

Physical Health

Over 80% (84.2%) of parents in the FNIRHS reported that their youth's (age 12 to 17) health was very good or excellent. Figure 6.1 shows the rates of medical conditions for FNIRHS youths, as reported by parents. Comparison figures for Canadian children aged newborn to 11 are available from the NLSCY Cycle 1; Cycle 3 data (children now aged 4 to 15) have been released but are not published.

One of the most prevalent chronic illnesses affecting Aboriginal people today is diabetes (Young, Szathmary, et al. 1990; Young, Schraer, et al. 1992; Young, Reading, et al. 2000); type 2 diabetes is increasingly recognized in Aboriginal youth (Canadian Pediatric Society Indian and Inuit Health Committee 1994). Among Aboriginal youths 15 to 24 years of age, 2.3% of males and 3.6% of females are diagnosed with diabetes, compared with 0.4% of the male and female Canadian youth population (Kidder et al. 2000). The Sandy Lake Health and Diabetes Project referred to above found no type 2 diabetes among males aged 10 to 19, but among females the rate was 40 per 1,000 (Harris et al. 1997; Fagot-Campagna et al. 2000). A Manitoba study found a similar prevalence of 36 per 1,000 for Aboriginal girls aged 10 to 19 years (Dean et al. 1998). The sex ratio is skewed, with 4 to 6 females affected for every male (Rosenbloom et al. 1999). Fagot-Campagna and colleagues (2000) argue that type 2 diabetes is a sizeable public health problem among American Indian and First Nations youth in the United States and Canada. As with adults, it appears closely linked to modifiable risk factors such as obesity, poor nutrition, and low physical activity (Fagot-Campagna et al. 2000; see Health Behaviours section above). Diabetes influences the emotional well-being of those affected and is associated with limitation in daily activity (First Nations and Inuit Regional Health Survey National Steering Committee 1999). There has been a recent

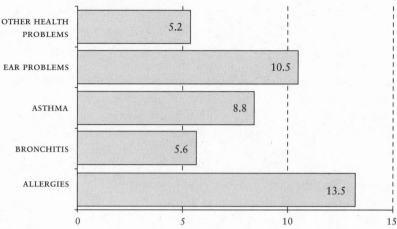

Figure 6.1
Prevalence of specified conditions in FNIRHS youth, parent report

emphasis on Aboriginal health promotion programs to increase physical activity and improve diet, but the long-term effectiveness of such strategies has not been established (Fagot-Campagna et al. 2000).

Aboriginal children and youth appear to be at increased risk for some infectious diseases such as lower respiratory tract infections (Fraser-Lee and Hessel 1994), hepatitis B, and otitis media, although the focus of these investigations has generally been on younger children (Harris et al. 1998). For example, based on the FNIRHS findings, the rate of bronchitis in Aboriginal children aged 0 to 5 years was 9% compared to 6% among those 12 years of age and older (MacMillan, Walsh, Jamieson, et al. 1999). It is not clear why Aboriginal people experience an increased risk of infectious diseases; some suggested correlates include poverty and overcrowding, nutritional problems, and environmental pollutants such as tobacco and wood smoke (MacMillan, MacMillan, et al. 1996).

Injuries are a major problem for Aboriginal young people, although death rates among First Nations youths 15 to 24 years of age as a result of some causes have declined recently (Kidder et al. 2000). The death rates related to motor vehicle injuries declined between the periods 1979 to 1983 and 1989 to 1993 from 87 to 62 per 100,000 population for this age group. Similarly, the drowning death rates declined from 25 to 9 per 100,000. In the FNIRHS, based on parental report, the lifetime prevalence of serious head injury was 4.6% for those 12 to 17 years of age; the rate for broken bones or fractures was 20.4% in this age group (MacMillan, Walsh, Jamieson, et al. 1999). The lifetime rate of serious burn injury was 4.2%, and for almost drowning it was 4.9%. Sample sizes were too small to report rates of frostbite or hypothermia in the 12– to 17–year age group, but the rate for all children was 2.0%. In the United States, American Indian and Alaska Native children and youth also experience higher rates of injury, morbidity, and mortality compared to their non-Native counterparts (American Academy of Pediatrics Committee on Native American Child Health and Committee on Injury and Poison Prevention 1999). This has led the American Academy of Pediatrics to advocate for a broad-based injury prevention program for Native children and youth.

One of the largest surveys assessing the health of American Native youth, the 1990 National American Indian Adolescent Health Survey, involved a sample of almost 13,500 reservation-based American Indian or Alaska Native students in grades 7 through 12 (Blum et al. 1992). While more than 78% of student respondents reported their health to be good or excellent, those who reported poor health showed an increase in risk of suicide attempts, substance abuse, and exposure to abuse. This underscores the importance of considering the relationship between physical health and psychosocial factors in Aboriginal youth.

Emotional Health

There are few Canadian data about the emotional health of Aboriginal youth. Since the FNIRHS included only ten core questions about child and youth health, the focus was predominantly on physical health; asking about emotional conditions such as anxiety or depression requires several questions for each problem. In response to a general question about the past six months, 23.4% of FNIRHS parents reported that their youth had emotional or behavioural problems. More in-depth questions in the NSFNRHS indicated that female youths were more than twice as likely to report being sad or depressed for at least two weeks in the year prior to the interview than were male youths (47% compared to 21%, respectively); however, OFNRHS parents reported that only 4.0% of youths had psychological problems. The OFNRHS has extensive information about the emotional health of children, but these data focus only on children 0 to 11 years of age (the reason being that information on this age group in the general population was available for comparison from the NLSCY).

One of the few studies to assess emotional health and academic achievement among a sample that included both American and Canadian Aboriginal young people was the Flower of Two Soils (FOTS) study (Beiser et al. 1998; Dion, Gotowiec, and Beiser 1998; Beiser, Dion, and Gotowiec 2000). This study included two cohorts of children in grades 2 and 4; the Canadian participants were living in parts of Manitoba and British Columbia. The mean age of the participants was 8 and 10 years, respectively, and so the latter group falls into the lower age range of what is considered adolescence. Despite previous literature showing that Native children and youth experience more psychopathology than do their non-Native peers, findings from the FOTS showed that self-ratings and parent ratings of depressive symptoms were higher for the majority-culture children than for their Native counterparts (Dion, Gotowiec, and Beiser 1998). Self- and parent ratings of conduct disorder were similar; only teachers tended to rate Native children higher on symptoms of conduct disorder and depression than their non-Native peers. This discrepancy suggests the possibility of a systematic bias in the way teachers assess Native children's behaviour.

A second important finding arising from the FOTS study related to differences in the way that Native and non-Native children perceived their competence to carry out school-related tasks (Beiser et al. 1998). While the two groups were comparable in grade 2, the self-concept of non-Native children became increasingly positive over time, whereas Native self-concepts became more negative. This was the case for both self-rated instrumental and social competence. Understanding the basis for these findings is important in assessing the ability of schools to meet the needs of Aboriginal children and youth.

The National American Indian Adolescent Health Survey included several items about emotional health (Blum et al. 1992; Cummins et al. 1999). It is important to highlight that the majority of American Indian-Alaska Native youths reported experiencing good emotional health, although a substantial minority reported stress and depression. Approximately 14% of females and 8.3% of males indicated feelings of sadness and hopelessness over the past month, and 5.7% reported symptoms of severe emotional distress. Factors associated with positive emotional health in female adolescents included perceived family caring, body pride, and a sense of connectedness to school (Cummins et al. 1999). For males, the strongest correlates with positive emotional health included perceived family caring, body pride, parental expectations, and a personal area of skill or competence. These factors are consistent with findings in the general resilience literature (Cummins et al. 1999).

This American study also examined the relationship between psychosocial factors and eating behaviours. Findings regarding concerns of Native American adolescents about weight control suggested that overweight youths are concerned about their weight but do not experience major psychosocial distress associated with being overweight (Neumark-Sztainer et al. 1997). Dieting and purging behaviours were, however, common among both males and females and were associated with health-risk behaviours such as substance abuse and suicide attempts (Story et al. 1997).

Each of the above studies assessed symptoms of emotional problems; there have been almost no epidemiological studies examining the presence of actual psychiatric disorders in Aboriginal youth (Beals et al. 1997). For example, while understanding whether youths experience feelings of sadness or worry is important, a crucial question is the extent to which they suffer from disorders associated with impairment requiring treatment. One recent American study is notable for having examined the presence of psychiatric disorders in a sample of Northern Plains youths between the ages of 14 and 16 (Beals et al. 1997). Within this group, the six-month prevalence rates were as follows: 10.6% for attention-deficit hyperactivity disorder, 3.8% for conduct disorder, 4.7% for major depressive disorder, and 18.3% for any substance abuse disorder. Although the sample included no non-Native comparison group, the findings provide important data about the mental health of American Indian adolescents. Unfortunately, no such Canadian data are available about the extent of these common conditions.

SUICIDE

I know all the reasons why I should not commit suicide. I know why I shouldn't take my own life. What I want to know is how not to commit suicide.

Aboriginal youth, Kingfisher Lake First Nation, Ontario, quoted in speech by Ovide Mercredi, National Chief, Assembly of First Nations (*Suicide Prevention Workshop* 1996, 20)

The suicide rate among Canadian Aboriginal youth continues to be alarmingly high; there is a fivefold increase among male Aboriginal youths and an eightfold increase among female Aboriginal youths compared to their counterparts in the total Canadian population (Kidder et al. 2000). This increase is recognized among First Nations youths (MacMillan, MacMillan, et al. 1996) as well as Inuit youths (Kirmayer, Boothroyd, and Hodgins 1998). Secondary analysis of data from a Santé Québec survey showed that 22% of the Inuit youth sample 15 to 24 years of age had attempted suicide (Kirmayer, Boothroyd, and Hodgins 1998). Multivariate analysis showed that, among females, attempted suicide was associated with psychiatric problems, alcohol abuse, and drug use, while the strongest correlates of attempted suicide for males were solvent use and a number of recent significant life events. Findings from the 1990 National American Indian Adolescent Health Survey provide important information about risk and protective factors for youth suicide (Borowsky et al. 1999). Increased risk of suicide attempts by both male and female youths was associated with friends or family members attempting or committing suicide, somatic symptoms, physical or sexual abuse, or substance abuse. Those factors associated with a reduced risk of suicide included discussing problems with friends or family members, good emotional health, and a sense of connectedness with family. These data, while useful, are based on a convenience sample of non-urban American Indian adolescents and therefore cannot be considered representative of the population of Native adolescents in the United States.

While suicide is clearly a major health issue among Aboriginal youth, using data based on British Columbia First Nations groups, Chandler and Lalonde (1998) emphasize that suicide rates vary widely. They highlight the fact that some communities show suicide rates up to eight hundred times the Canadian average, whereas suicide is essentially unknown in other communities. The authors suggest that risk of suicide among First Nations youth is heightened for those "who have lost a sense of connectedness to their own future" (198). They refer to research showing that actively suicidal adolescents differ from their non-suicidal counterparts in their inability to understand themselves as continuous in time – a concept the authors refer to as self-continuity. Chandler and Lalonde explore the links between self-continuity and cultural continuity to determine those cultural factors that appear to protect youths from the risk of suicide within First Nations communities. In an attempt to operationalize cultural continuity, they identified the following markers of cultural continuity: (a) evidence that bands were working on securing title to their traditional lands, (b) evidence of seeking self-government, (c) indication of some community control over educational services, (d) police and fire services, (e) health delivery services, and (f) evidence of having established certain cultural facilities within communities. Each of these six markers of cultural continuity was associated with a "clinically important reduction in the rate of youth suicide" (215). For example, when all six of these factors were in place, the observed five-year suicide rate was zero, whereas in those communities in which none of the factors was present, the youth suicide rate was 137.5 per 100,000. These findings suggest that rates of youth suicides among First Nations communities are strongly linked to a group of factors that measure the degree to which communities are involved in efforts to "preserve and restore their Native culture" (213).

The work of Chandler and Lalonde (1998) examining connections between self- and cultural continuity is highlighted in this chapter because of its contribution to new knowledge in the area of Aboriginal youth health and its potential for feasible solutions. As the authors state, each of these factors represents an aspect over which a community can exert some control. In their paper, they point to the futility of repeatedly advising First Nations people that youth suicide is directly linked only to impoverished living conditions. It is also crucial to underscore the fact that youth suicide is not a problem in some First Nations communities.

Several groups have made recommendations regarding the problem of suicide among Aboriginal people, including RCAP (RCAP 1995). In its *Special Report on Suicide*, RCAP argued that only a comprehensive approach to suicide prevention will improve the situation in Aboriginal communities. Such an approach includes: "plans and programs that provide suicide crisis services, promote broad preventive action and community development, and address long-term needs for self-determination, self-sufficiency, and healing" (RCAP 1995, 75). While not specific to youth, the guidelines outlined by Kirmayer, Boothroyd, and colleagues (1999) suggest a suicide prevention program that is likely to be effective in Native communities. Ideally, a suicide prevention program for Aboriginal communities would meet the following criteria: have proven effectiveness, reach high-risk groups, be feasible given local resources, and address both immediate and basic long-term causes. To date no such programs have been demonstrated to be effective in preventing suicide, but there are some promising programs that deserve further evaluation (Kirmayer, Boothroyd, et al. 1999). The RCAP report provides case studies of five programs that serve to highlight activities that contribute to successful mental health promotion strategies among Aboriginal people. The activities were community-initiated, drew upon traditional knowledge and wisdom of elders, were based on consultation with the community, and were broad in focus. Most involved locally controlled partnerships with external groups. The programs emphasized that strategies aimed at community and social development should promote community pride and control; self-esteem and identity; transmission of Aboriginal knowledge, language, and traditions; and culturally appropriate methods of addressing social problems (Kirmayer, Hayton, et al. 1993; RCAP 1995).

Clearly, there is an urgent need for rigorous evaluation in this area; the recent United States Surgeon General's report on suicide prevention (Surgeon General 2001), while not specific to Aboriginal youth, noted the absence of evaluation research indicating which methods of suicide prevention are effective. The lack of information is even more marked for Aboriginal people, including youths, who represent one of the highest risk groups. In July 2001, an advisory group on suicide prevention was convened by Health Canada and the Assembly of First Nations. This group was given the task of making recommendations to address the issue of youth suicide among the First Nations in Canada, based on review of previous studies and recommendations regarding suicide prevention. The recommendations of this advisory group should be available in 2002.

Social Health

Based on parental reports regarding youth, the rate of frequent or constant problems for youths in their social relationships with friends or classmates was higher in females (6.6%) than males (1.0%), as illustrated in Figure 6.2. This was also true in social relationships with teachers, where the proportion was 13.8% of females compared with 4.7% of males. Of note, parents also reported that 67.4% of youths get along very well or quite well with their family. A higher percentage of male youths than of female youths

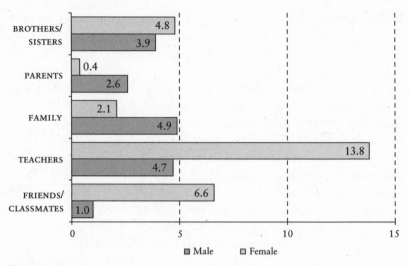

Figure 6.2
Frequent or constant problems in social relationships, by gender,
from OFNRHS youth self-report

was identified as having frequent or constant problems with the family. Results from the NSFNRHS, based on youth self-report, showed a different pattern from that of the OFNRHS; a higher proportion of females than males had problems getting along in their families (9% of females versus 2% of males reported getting along "not well at all" with the family).

A great majority of OFNRHS youth respondents (84.8%) indicated that their parents take "care of me." Similarly, 78.3% reported that their caretaker "makes me feel I am loved." With regard to a question about whether caretakers "don't care where I am," 21.4% reported that this occurred often or very often. Almost 11% of youths indicated that their parents "call me things like stupid, lazy or ugly" often or very often.

Very little information regarding sexual relationships is available. A survey of 3,040 students in grades 7 to 10 in the Northwest Territories in 1994 showed that 24% to 27% of Aboriginal youths (Dene, Métis, or Inuit) in grades 7 to 8 have had sexual intercourse at least once, compared to 12% in the non-Aboriginal sample. Similarly, rates for Aboriginal students in grades 9 to 10 were 56% to 68% compared with 35% for non-Aboriginals. Of those who reported having sex "often," Dene and Inuit students were less likely to have protected sexual intercourse than were Métis and non-Aboriginal students (Peart and King 1996).

Hopes and Dreams

When, through an open-ended question, OFNRHS adolescents were asked about their hopes and dreams for the future, they suggested that education and employment opportunities were paramount. Education was rated as important for 37.9% of the youths, followed by employment (34.8%) and a successful career (26%). Other factors that were important for the future of youths included their family (17.9%), maintaining their culture (12.7%), athletic activities (10.4%), happiness (9.5%), and, finally, health (4.2%). In reporting their concerns for their family, youths were most concerned about happiness (57.4%), health (27.2%), and finances (12.8%).

Adolescents were also asked to provide information about their hopes and dreams for their community. Forty-five percent of respondents wanted improvements in their community, 25.4% hoped for prosperity, and a further 21.4% felt that maintaining the First Nations culture was important for their community. The next most frequent suggestions for the future of the community were survival (16.0%) and happiness (14.8%). In an open-ended question, youths were also asked about their opportunities or plans to contribute to their community. Although more than half (51.8%) of the respondents said they could contribute through sharing their knowledge and skills, and a further 32.1% felt that they could improve their community, 8.9% believed that they had no opportunities or plans to contribute to their community.

FUTURE DIRECTIONS

The ability of Aboriginal youth to meet the challenge of coping with the divergence between traditional culture and modern mainstream society, while maintaining their connectedness with community and culture, has implications for their futures, including educational and employment opportunities. There is a sense of hope for the present and future of Aboriginal youth that has been demonstrated by positive Aboriginal role models who have received exposure in both the Aboriginal community and mainstream media across Canada. There are many initiatives at the community, regional, and national levels that are beginning to recognize the considerable achievements of Aboriginal youth. In Aboriginal culture, there is the "seven generations" concept: what is accomplished in this life-time has future implications as far as seven generations. The collec-tive will of Aboriginal and mainstream society, including individuals, the social service and health care systems, and all levels of govern-ment, to meaningfully address the issues outlined in this chapter regarding Aboriginal youth can have an influence on this concept. Aboriginal youths may be strengthened in their physical, mental, emotional, and spiritual aspects so that they can provide a substan-tial, vital, and durable foundation for the future of Aboriginal peoples in this country.

While it is tempting to make broad recommendations regarding issues such as the need to improve the life quality of Aboriginal youths, we want to avoid the long-standing pattern of authors' putting forth beliefs about Aboriginal needs and goals, when it is the responsibility of Aboriginal people to do so in order to further their self-determina-tion as a people. Nonetheless, this chapter identifies considerable gaps in knowledge regarding the health of Canadian Aboriginal youth. There is an urgent need for information about the following:

(a) risk and protective factors at the individual and community levels regarding the physical, emotional, and social health of Aboriginal youths;
(b) rigorous evaluations of any programs or interventions that purport to improve the health of Aboriginal youths; and
(c) evaluation of the impact on Aboriginal youths of broad-based initiatives such as community development, land claims, and governmental policies (e.g., the implementation of self-government among Aboriginal communities).

Many of the sections in this chapter rely heavily on information from American Native youth groups because comparable Canadian data are not available. Development of meaningful policy recom-mendations is dependent on the availability of valid information about the status and determinants of health of Aboriginal youths in Canada. Furthermore, there are very few data about regional differ-ences suitable for comparison. Even the OFNRHS and NSFNRHS have substantive differences in the actual questions included in their respective survey instruments. This underscores the need for careful consideration of issues such as sampling, measurement, and other aspects of methodology for future regional and national surveys involving Aboriginal youths.

It is hoped that the information summarized in this chapter will be useful to Aboriginal communities, organizations, and policy-makers in determining approaches to improve the life quality and health of Aboriginal youth.

REFERENCES

Adlaf, E.M., A. Paglia, F.J. Ivis, and A. Ialomiteanu. 2000. Nonmedical drug use among adolescent students: Highlights from the 1999 Ontario Student Drug Use Survey. *Canadian Medical Association Journal* 162(12):1677–80.

American Academy of Pediatrics Committee on Native American Child Health and Committee on Injury and Poison Prevention. 1999. The prevention of unintentional injury among American Indian and Alaska Native children: A subject review. *Pediatrics* 104:1397–99.

Assembly of First Nations. 1998. *Residential School Update*. Cornwall, ON: Assembly of First Nations Health Secretariat.

Beals, J., J. Piasecki, S. Nelson, M. Jones, E. Keane, P. Dauphinais, R.R. Shirt, W.H. Sack, and S.M. Manson. 1997. Psychiatric disorder among American Indian adolescents: Prevalence in Northern Plains youth. *Journal of the American Academy of Child and Adolescent Psychiatry* 36:1252–59.

Beiser, M. 1981. Mental health of American Indian and Alaska Native children: Some epidemiologic perspectives. *White Cloud Journal* 2:37–47.

Beiser, M., R. Dion, and A. Gotowiec. 2000. The structure of attention-deficit and hyperactivity symptoms among native and non-native elementary school children. *Journal of Abnormal Child Psychology* 28:425–37.

Beiser, M., W. Sack, S.M. Manson, R. Redshirt, and R. Dion. 1998. Mental health and the academic performance of first nations and majority-culture children. *American Journal of Orthopsychiatry* 68:455–67.

Blum, R.W., B. Harmon, L. Harris, L. Bergeisen, and M.D. Resnick. 1992. American Indian-Alaska Native youth health. *Journal of the American Medical Association* 267:1637–44.

Borowsky, I.W., M.D. Resnick, M. Ireland, and R.W. Blum. 1999. Suicide attempts among American Indian and Alaska Native youth: Risk and protective factors. *Archives of Pediatric and Adolescent Medicine* 153:573–80.

Bray, D.L., and P.D. Anderson. 1989. Appraisal of the epidemiology of fetal alcohol syndrome among Canadian native peoples. *Canadian Journal of Public Health* 80:42–5.

Burd, L., and M.E. Moffatt. 1994. Epidemiology of fetal alcohol syndrome in American Indians, Alaskan Natives, and Canadian Aboriginal peoples: A review of the literature. *Public Health Reports* 109:688–93.

Canadian Pediatric Society Indian and Inuit Health Committee. Diabetes and the first nations. *Canadian Journal of Paediatrics* 1:222–5.

Chandler, M.J., and C. Lalonde. 1998. Cultural continuity as a hedge against suicide in Canada's First Nations. *Transcultural Psychiatry* 35:191–219.

Cummins, J.R., M. Ireland, M.D. Resnick, and R.W. Blum. 1999. Correlates of physical and emotional health among Native American adolescents. *Journal of Adolescent Health* 24:38–44.

Dean, H.J., T.K. Young, B. Flett, and P. Wood-Steinman. 1998. Screening for non-type 2 diabetes in Aboriginal children in northern Canada [letter]. *Lancet* 39:1523–4.

Dewailly, E., P. Ayotte, S. Bruneau, C. Laliberte, D.C.G. Muir, and R.J. Norstrom. 1993. Inuit exposure to organochlorines through the aquatic food chain in arctic Quebec. *Environmental Health Perspective* 101:618–20.

Dickason, O.M. 1997. *Canada's First Nations: A History of the Founding Peoples from the Earliest Times*, 2nd ed. Toronto: Oxford University Press.

Dion, R., A. Gotowiec, and M. Beiser. 1998. Depression and conduct disorder in native and non-native children. *Journal of the American Academy of Child and Adolescent Psychiatry* 37:736–42.

Fagot-Campagna, A., D.J. Pettitt, M.M. Engelgau, N. Riios Burrows, J. Saaddine, J. Geiss, R. Valdez, G. Beckles, E.W. Gregg, D.F. Williamson, and K.M.V. Narayan. 2000. Type 2 diabetes among North American children and adolescents: An epidemiologic review and a public health perspective. *Journal of Pediatrics* 136:664–72.

Federal, Provincial, and Territorial Advisory Committee on Population Health. 1999. *Towards a Healthy Future: Second Report on the Health of Canadians*. Health Canada Catalogue #H39–468/1999E. Ottawa: Minister of Public Works and Government Services.

First Nations and Inuit Regional Health Survey National Steering Committee. 1999. *First Nations and Inuit Regional Health Survey: National Report*. Ottawa: First Nations and Inuit Regional Health Survey National Steering Committee.

Fournier, S., and E. Crey. 1997. *Stolen from Our Embrace: The Abduction of First Nations and the Restoration of Aboriginal Communities*. Vancouver: Douglas and McIntyre.

Fraser-Lee, N.J., and P.A. Hessel. 1994. Acute respiratory infections in the Canadian native Indian population: A review. *Canadian Journal of Public Health* 85:197–200.

Gfellner, B.M., and J.D. Hundleby. 1995. Patterns of drug use among native and white adolescents: 1990–1993. *Canadian Journal of Public Health* 86:95–7.

Guo, S.S., A.F. Roche, W.C. Chumlea, J.D. Gardner, and R.M. Siervogel. 1994. The predictive value of childhood body mass index values for overweight at age 35 years. *American Journal of Clinical Nutrition* 59:810–19.

Hanley, A.J.G., S.B. Harris, J. Gittelsohn, T.M.S. Wikever, B. Saksvig, and B. Zinman. 2000. Overweight among children and adolescents in a Native Canadian community: Prevalence and associated factors. *American Journal of Clinical Nutrition* 71:693–700.

Hanvey, Louise. 1994. Aboriginal children. In *The Health of Canada's Children: A CICH Profile*, 2nd ed., 131–48. Ottawa: Canadian Institute of Child Health.

Harris, S.B., J. Gittelsohn, A. Hanley, A. Barnie, T.M. Wolever, J. Gao, A. Logan, and B. Zinman. 1997. The prevalence of NIDDM and associated risk factors in native Canadians. *Diabetes Care* 20:185–7.

Harris, S.B., R. Glazier, K. Eng, and L. McMurray. 1998. Disease patterns among Canadian aboriginal children: Study in a remote rural setting. *Canadian Family Physician* 44:1869–77.

Hoover, J., R. McDermott, and T. Hartsfield. 1990. The prevalence of smokeless tobacco use in native children in northern Saskatchewan, Canada. *Canadian Journal of Public Health* 81:350–2.

Human Resources Development Canada (HRDC) and Statistics Canada. 1996. *Growing Up in Canada: National Longitudinal Survey of Children and Youth*. Ottawa: Statistics Canada.

Johnston, B. 1982. *Ojibway Ceremonies*. Lincoln, NE: University of Nebraska Press.

Kidder, Karen, J. Stein, J. Fraser, and G. Chance. 2000. Aboriginal children and youth. In *The Health of Canada's Children: A CICH Profile*, 3rd ed., 143–76. Ottawa: Canadian Institute of Child Health.

King, A.J.C., W.F. Boyce, and M.A. King. 1999. *Trends in the Health of Canadian Youth: Health Behaviour in School-aged Children*. Catalogue #H39–498/1999E. Ottawa: Health Canada.

Kirmayer, L.J., L.J. Boothroyd, and S. Hodgins. 1998. Attempted suicide among Inuit youth: Psychosocial correlates and implications for prevention. *Canadian Journal of Psychiatry* 43:816–22.

Kirmayer, L.J., L.J. Boothroyd, A. Laliberté, and B. Laronde Simpson. 1999. *Suicide prevention and mental health promotion in Native communities* (Working Paper No. 9). Montreal, QC: Culture and Mental Health Research Unit, Institute of Community and Family Psychiatry, Sir Mortimer B. Davis Jewish General Hospital.

Kirmayer, L.J., G.M. Brass, and C.L. Tait. 2000. The mental health of Aboriginal peoples: Transformations of identity and community. *Canadian Journal of Psychiatry* 45:607–16.

Kirmayer, L.J., B.C. Hayton, M. Malus, W. Jimenez, R. Dufour, C. Quesney, Y. Ternar, T. Yu, and N. Ferrarra. 1993. *Suicide in Canadian Aboriginal Populations: Emerging Trends in Research and Clinical Intervention*. Montreal, Quebec: Culture and Mental Health Research Unit, Department of Psychiatry, Sir Mortimer B. Davis Jewish General Hospital.

Lalinec-Michaud, M., M.E. Subak, A.M. Ghadirian, and V. Kovess. 1991. Substance misuse among native and rural high school students in Quebec. *International Journal of Addiction* 26:1003–12.

Lanier, A.P., L.R. Bulkow, T.E. Novotny, G.A. Giovino, and R.M. Davis. 1990. Tobacco use and its consequences in northern populations. *Arctic Medical Research* 49:17–22.

Mackie, Richard. 2002. Walkerton final report urges fast action to safeguard water. *Globe and Mail*, 24 May, A1.

MacMillan, H.L., J.E. Fleming, N. Trocme, M.H. Boyle, M. Wong, Y.A. Racine, W.R. Beardslee, and D.R. Offord. 1997. Prevalence of child physical and sexual abuse in the community. *Journal of the American Medical Association* 278(2):131–5.

MacMillan, H.L., A.B. MacMillan, D.R. Offord, and J.L. Dingle. 1996. Aboriginal health. *Canadian Medical Association Journal* 155:1569–78.

MacMillan, H.L., C. Walsh, E. Faries, A.B. MacMillan, H. McCue, M. Wong, D. Offord, and Technical Advisory Committee, Chiefs of Ontario. 1998. Ontario First Nations Regional Health Survey: Final Report.

MacMillan, H.L., C. Walsh, E. Jamieson, A. Crawford, and M. Boyle. 1999. Children's health. In *First Nations and Inuit Regional Health Survey: National Report*, 1–26. Ottawa: First Nations and Inuit Regional Health Survey National Steering Committee.

Metler, R., G.A. Conway, and J. Stehr-Green. 1991. AIDS surveillance among American Indians and Alaska natives. *American Journal of Public Health* 81:1469–71.

Mi'kmaq Health Research Group. 1999. *The Health of the Nova Scotia Mi'kmaq Population: A Final Research Report.* Sydney, NS: Mi'kmaq Health Research Group.

Millar, W.J. 1990a. Smoking prevalence in the Canadian Arctic. *Arctic Medical Research* 49(suppl 2):23–28.

– 1990b. Smokeless tobacco use by youth in the Canadian Arctic. *Arctic Medical Research* 49(suppl 2):39–47.

Moffatt, M.E. 1995. Current status of nutritional deficiencies in Canadian aboriginal people. *Canadian Journal of Physiology and Pharmacology* 73:754–8.

Muir, B.L. 1988. *Health Status of Canadian Indians and Inuit: Update 1987.* Ottawa: Medical Services Branch, Department of National Health and Welfare.

Neumark-Sztainer, D., M. Story, M.D. Resnick, and R.W. Blum. 1997. Psychosocial concerns and weight control behaviors among overweight and nonoverweight Native American adolescents. *Journal of the American Dietetic Association* 6:598–604.

Ng, E. 1996. Disability among Canada's aboriginal peoples in 1991. *Health Reports* 8(1):25–32 (Eng); 25–33 (Fre).

Novins, D.K., J. Beals, and C.M. Mitchell. 2001. Sequences of substance use among American Indian adolescents. *Journal of the American Academy of Child and Adolescent Psychiatry* 40:1168–74.

Offord, D.R., D. Cadman, I. Antone, C. George, and J. McNamee. 1989. *First Nations Child Health Care Study: Final Report.* Toronto: Ministry of Community and Social Services.

Peart, M.J., and A.J.C. King. 1996. *Health Behaviours, Attitudes and Knowledge of Young People in the Northwest Territories.* Northwest Territories Department of Education, Culture and Employment.

Pickering, J., C. Lavallee, and J. Hanley. 1989. Cigarette smoking in Cree Indian school children of the James Bay region. *Arctic Medical Research* 48:6–11.

Postl, B. 1997. It's time for action: The underserved and desperate: Native health. *Canadian Medical Association Journal* 157:1655–6.

Postl, B., J. Irvine, S. MacDonald, and M. Moffatt. 1994. Background paper on the health of aboriginal peoples in Canada. In *Bridging the Gap: Promoting Health and Healing for Aboriginal Peoples in Canada*, 19–56. Ottawa: Canadian Medical Association.

Potthoff, S.J., L.H. Bearinger, C.L. Skay, N. Cassuto, R.W. Blum, and M.D. Resnick. 1998. Dimensions of risk behaviors among American Indian youth. *Archives of Pediatric and Adolescent Medicine* 152:157–63.

Remington, G., and B.F. Hoffman. 1984. Gas sniffing as a form of substance abuse. *Canadian Journal of Psychiatry* 29:31–5.

Rosenbloom, A.L., J.R. Joe, R.S. Young, and W.E. Winter. 1999. Emerging epidemic of type 2 diabetes in youth. *Diabetes Care* 22:345–354.

Royal Commission on Aboriginal Peoples (RCAP). 1995. *Choosing Life: Special Report on Suicide among Aboriginal People.* Ottawa: Canada Communication Group.

Starkey, L.J., L. Johnson-Down, and K. Gray-Donald. 2001. Food habits of Canadians: Comparison of intakes in adults and adolescents to Canada's food guide to healthy eating. *Canadian Journal of Dietary Practice and Research* 62(2):61–69.

Statistics Canada. 1991. *Language, Tradition, Health, Lifestyle and Social Issues: 1991 Aboriginal Peoples Survey.* Catalogue #89–533. Ottawa: Statistics Canada.

– 1992. *1991 Census of Canada.* Catalogue #93–310. Ottawa: Statistics Canada.

– 1993a. *1991 Census of Canada.* Catalogue #94–327. Ottawa: Statistics Canada.

– 1993b. *Schooling, Work and Related Activities, Income, Expenses and Mobility: 1991 Aboriginal Peoples Survey.* Catalogue #89–534. Ottawa: Statistics Canada.

– 1996. *1996 Census of Canada.* Ottawa: Statistics Canada.

Story, M., F.R. Hauck, B.A. Broussard, L.L. White, M.D. Resnick, and R.W. Blum. 1994. Weight perceptions and weight control practices in American Indian and Alaska Native adolescents: A national survey. *Archives of Pediatric and Adolescent Medicine* 148:567–71.

Stout, M.D., and G.D. Kipling. 1999. Emerging priorities for the health of First Nations and Inuit children and youth. Draft discussion paper prepared for the Strategic Policy, Planning, and Analysis Directorate, First Nations and Inuit Health Branch (FNIHB), 30 November.

Suicide Prevention Workshop: Framework for Living. 1996. Proceedings of the workshop, London, Ontario, 1995. Ottawa: Health Canada, Medical Services Branch, Brighter Futures Initiative.

Surgeon General. 2001. *National Strategy for Suicide Prevention: Goals and Objectives for Action.* Rockville, MD: US Department of Health and Human Services.

Waldram, J.B., D.A. Herring, and T.K. Young. 1995. *Aboriginal Health in Canada: Historical, Cultural and Epidemiological Perspectives.* Toronto: University of Toronto Press.

Webster, S.T. 2000. The health and well-being of Aboriginal children and youth. In *The Health of Canada's Children: A CICH Profile*, 3rd ed., 144–145. Ottawa: Canadian Institute of Child Health.

Young, T.K., J. Reading, B. Elias, and J.D. O'Neil. 2000. Type 2 diabetes mellitus in Canada's First Nations: Status of an epidemic in progress. *Canadian Medical Association Journal* 163:561–6.

Young, T.K., C.D. Schraer, E.V. Shubnikoff, E.J.E. Szathmary, and Y.P. Nikitin. 1992. Prevalence of diagnosed diabetes in circumpolar indigenous populations. *International Journal of Epidemiology* 21:730–6.

Young, T.K., E.J.E. Szathmary, S. Evers, and B. Wheatley. 1990. Geographical distribution of diabetes among the native population of Canada: A national survey. *Social Science and Medicine* 31:129–39.

7

Sexuality and Reproductive Health in Adolescence: Policy Implications of Early Age of Sexual Debut

ROGER S. TONKIN, AILEEN MURPHY,
AND COLLEEN S. POON

INTRODUCTION

Although adolescence may be difficult to define, it is clear that certain developmental tasks take place within the adolescent period. The development of secondary sex characteristics and the emergence of sexual identity are cornerstones of the developmental tasks of adolescence (*Adolescent Medicine* 1991). How youths confront these challenges can become important correlates of their emerging sexuality. As Rutter notes, "Sexuality is very important to adolescents and much talk centres around the topic" (1979, 16).

These tasks are not achieved in isolation from the other developmental challenges of the period. Cognitive capacity, emotional development, lifestyle choices, peer and other social relationships, and connectedness to school and family are but a few of the critical determinants of adolescent sexual and reproductive health. As the World Health Organization (WHO) and some US-based authorities such as the National Commission on Adolescent Sexual Health have reported, these determinants must be considered when formulating national social policy, drafting legislation, or designing programs to address adolescent reproductive health in both developed and developing countries (Alan Guttmacher Institute 1998; Annie E. Casey Foundation 1998; Senderowitz 1997).

In 1985, the WHO authored a position paper entitled "Reproductive Health in Adolescence." This was one of the earliest reports to address the issues of global policy on behalf of reproductive health in adolescence. While its focus was almost entirely on early child-bearing in developing nations, the WHO paper linked the challenge of addressing this pressing issue with the opportunity for placing its solutions in the context of healthy adolescent development. A decade later, the US National Commission on Adolescent Sexual Health released a consensus statement that further shifted the emphasis beyond pregnancy prevention and the avoidance of contracting sexually transmitted diseases (STDs) to the notion that becoming a sexually healthy adult is a key developmental task for adolescents (Haffner 1995). In this chapter, sexuality and reproductive health issues are considered as two interrelated aspects of normal adolescent development, and reproductive health care is discussed within the context of the full spectrum of reproductive services, from health promotion to disease prevention, treatment, and follow-up care.

The United Nations Convention on the Rights of the Child (UNCRC) is an important vehicle for challenging governments to address the underlying principles of individual rights for children, including adolescents (United Nations 1989). Its various articles contain language that can be used to guide and subsequently evaluate policy frameworks and programs. While the Convention seems more relevant to the early childhood focus of Canada's National Children's Agenda, it does embrace the middle childhood and adolescent phases. Based on the policy implications of the Convention, it can be argued that early intervention in adolescence should itself become a national priority rather than a minor issue incorporated within the National Children's Agenda (Tonkin 1997, 2001b, in press). Evidence is presented here to document the special vulnerabilities and risks to reproductive health that occur in early adolescence. Several articles of the Convention on the Rights of the Child have particular relevance in this regard. These include Articles 13 (freedom to seek information), 16 (protection of privacy), 17 (access to information), 19 (protection), 23 (disability), 24 (health, treatment, rehabilitation), 25 (review of treatment for those in care), 32 (workplace protection), 33 (protection from substance abuse), 34 (protection from sexual exploitation/abuse), and 39 (treatment and recovery from abuse). Overall, however, the rights of adolescents and the specific issues of adolescent sexuality and reproductive health are poorly addressed in the Convention.

Canada has neither national nor provincial youth health policies that can be applied to adolescent sexual and reproductive health

(Rodriguez-Garcia et al. 2000). Essential issues in current Canadian policy and legislation include the need for: accessible, adolescent-friendly reproductive health services; dissemination of clearly expressed clinical guidelines and practices with respect to confidentiality; access to factual information and sexual health education; adequately funded research on adolescent sexual health and evaluation of programs; and better opportunities for meaningful youth participation in shaping sexual and reproductive health policies. Of course, it would be helpful to young Canadians and policy-makers if the language of the Convention were more explicit on adolescent themes.[1] These include, for example, reproductive health care issues such as: age of consent to sex, age of consent to treatment, reporting duties of professionals, the rights of parents when adolescents begin to engage in risky behaviours, and the role of community agencies vis-à-vis promotion of safe sex practices. In the absence of such international guidelines, this chapter focuses on sexual and reproductive health for Canadian adolescents and on related policies, programs, and legislation in Canada. The emphasis is on early adolescence, sexual debut, and exploitation/abuse. Wherever possible, issues are discussed in the context of available Canadian evidence, focusing particularly on research in British Columbia.

THE CURRENT STATE OF KNOWLEDGE ON ADOLESCENT SEXUAL HEALTH

Overall, the profile of the sexual and reproductive health of Canadian youth compares favourably with that of most other nations. Pregnancy, live-birth rates, and abortions among 15– to 19–year-olds are comparable to those of other developed nations and have declined in the past two decades. Maternal mortality is rare, and the prevalence of STDs and HIV/AIDS among adolescents is relatively low (Kidder, Stein, and Fraser 2000; see also Tables 7.1 and 7.2).[2] Important exceptions are increasing rates for chlamydia, which can lead to pelvic inflammatory disease and infertility, and human papillomavirus (HPV), which can lead to cervical cancer (Patrick, Wong, and Jordan 2000). Low rates for these negative outcomes are reflective of delays in sexual debut and the infrequency of sexual intercourse among otherwise sexually active adolescents. Sexual debut is defined by an affirmative answer by students to the survey question "Have you ever had sexual intercourse (gone all the way)?" It is

Table 7.1
Pregnancy rate and outcomes among Canadian females aged 15–19 years

Pregnancy rate	42.7 per 1,000
Live births	20.0 per 1,000
Abortions	22.0 per 1,000

Source: Statistics Canada. 1998. *Survey of Consumer Finances 1998: Individuals, Aged 15 Years and Over, With and Without Income, 1997 Income.* Public-use microdata file. Ottawa: Statistics Canada. [Results of the National Population Health Survey, Cycle 2, 1996/97.]

Table 7.2
STD rates among Canadian youths aged 15–19 years

STD	RATE PER 100,000
Chlamydia:	
Female	1255.1
Male	233.8
Gonorrhea:	
Female	97.9
Male	42.9
Syphilis:	
Female	1.0
Male	0.4

Source: Public Health Agency of Canada. N.d. 2002 *Canadian Sexually Transmitted Infections (STI) Surveillance Report.* Pre-release. http://www.phac-aspc.gc.ca/std-mts/stddata_pre06_04/index.html#tables. Retrieved 8 February 2005.

recognized, however, that adolescents become sexually active without actually engaging in what is traditionally defined as sexual intercourse. Alternative forms of sexual activity might include mutual masturbation, oral or anal sex, and expressions of homosexual orientation. Of the total population of 15- to 19–year-old high school students in British Columbia, only 35% report having ever had sexual intercourse (McCreary Centre Society 1999a). This rate is lower than what is reported in a number of European countries and the United States (Currie et al. 2001). The low rate of exposure to risk and the ease of access to reproductive care are major factors in the current excellent sexual and reproductive health status of adolescents in Canada.

Social and individual attitudes towards sexual activity can vary over time. In British Columbia during the 1990s, the proportion of sexually active high school students declined from 30% in 1992 to

24% in 1998 (McCreary Centre Society 1999b). American studies indicate a similar decrease in sexual activity among adolescents (Centers for Disease Control and Prevention 2001). The reasons for this change are not well understood but may be related to adolescents' concerns for their health (e.g., preventing HIV/AIDS) or for their academic prospects (e.g., avoiding pregnancy). Whatever the underlying reasons for a decrease in sexual activity, the data are encouraging because they provide evidence that adolescent behaviour is changeable.

There are important differences, however, in the sexual behaviours of adolescents based on location and gender. Urban adolescents have lower pregnancy rates, lower birth rates, and a higher rate of terminated pregnancies than do non-urban adolescent populations (British Columbia Provincial Health Officer 1996). Gender plays an important role in any paradigm of adolescent sexuality and reproductive health, and emerging research based on feminist principles has particular importance to our understanding of sexuality and positive sexual health among early adolescent females (Tolman 1999). For recent information on adolescent males and their issues, the reader is referred to the World Health Organization publication *What about Boys?* (Barker 2000). Unfortunately, overall indicators of sexual health are of limited utility when considering high-risk populations of youths. In British Columbia, for example, only 12% of sexually active youths attending school report having contracted an STD or becoming pregnant, as compared to 42% of sexually active street youths (McCreary Centre Society 2001a).

A number of studies have been undertaken to provide a better knowledge base of adolescent health and behaviour in Canada. The best known is the Health Behaviours in School-aged Children (HBSC), the WHO cross-national study involving Europe and North America (King, Boyce, and King 1999). The HBSC provides important information on health trends of Canadian youths but contains no data on the sexual and reproductive health of Canada's adolescents until the 2001–2002 version. This limitation of the HBSC has been partially compensated for by other national and provincial studies (Bibby 2001; Langille et al. 1998; Statistics Canada 1998; Thomas, DiCenso, and Griffith 1998a, 1998b). The *Canada Youth and AIDS Study* (King et al.1988) is another resource regarding adolescent sexual health, and its results are being updated through the current school-based *Canadian Youth, Sexual Health, and HIV/AIDS Study*

(Boyce et al. 2003). Most of these studies use survey methodology and are population-based.

Other reports offer a compendium of data drawn from extant sources, such as vital statistics, hospitalization data, or population-based surveys of individuals over 15 years (Kidder, Stein, and Fraser 2000). The utility of these data sets for adolescent health policy, however, is compromised because of underreporting of abortions and STDs, failure to include adolescents under 15 years, and the common practice of releasing data for a combined 15– to 24–year age group. Despite these limitations, the available research data could be useful in informing national or provincial policy. Much of this data was reviewed by Godin and Michaud (1998) as part of their chapter "STD and AIDS prevention among young people" for the National Forum on Health.

Adolescent- or youth-specific health research generally has been a low priority among researchers in Canada. Research efforts often have been limited by lack of fiscal and human resources and by community and school resistance to asking young people about their health and behaviours (Tonkin 2001a). Most research has been either clinical or population-based and has not been clearly linked to youth-specific programs, policy, or legislation. Since most adolescent surveys do not include out-of-school youths and fail to cover all dimensions of adolescent behaviour, they cannot provide a comprehensive picture of adolescent health. Researchers may choose to not incorporate items on sensitive issues, such as sexual orientation or abuse, or may sacrifice full regional coverage in favour of cheaper, more convenient urban-based sampling strategies. Important regional differences in adolescent health resulting from north-south or rural-urban gradients in reproductive health care often are missed, and special populations are ignored. These deficiencies perpetuate myths about sexual health and represent significant information gaps with respect to important determinants of adolescent sexuality.

In the past decade and a half, the McCreary Centre Society, a British Columbia-based youth health organization, has conducted omnibus-type surveys of adolescent health and risk behaviour. The Adolescent Health Surveys (AHS) use a confidential, quantitative, self-report questionnaire format. These include province-wide sampling of grades 7 to 12 students as well as convenience samples of special populations, such as street youth and gay, lesbian, bisexual, transgender, and questioning (GLBTQ) youth. In the absence of a comprehensive, standardized, population-based, and regionally relevant strategy for surveying adolescent health status and risk behaviour on which to anchor an evidence-based policy, the remainder of this chapter continues to rely on data from British Columbia. While limited to a single province, the AHS surveys are sufficiently broad in terms of age range, regional representation, and topics to enable their use as the primary evidence base for the remaining discussion of policy, program, and legislation issues in this chapter.

EARLY SEXUAL MATURATION

While sexual identity formation is a deeply personal experience and is closely linked to exploring the dimensions of intimacy in relationships, it evolves in close connection with the timing of puberty. Tanner (1978) has documented the considerable range in ages and stages of pubertal change. This variability is most noticeable in early adolescence. The entry into adolescence can be more difficult for those who mature earlier or later than average (Rutter 1979). Timing of puberty may influence emotional and social development or contribute to emotionally influenced problems, such as eating disorders (Kaltiala-Heino et al. 2001).

Over the past century, the average age of onset of puberty has advanced by about three years (Rutter 1979). This is best documented in females, but evidence indicates similar changes for males. Reasons for this change may include better nutrition, better health (possibly lower rates of infectious diseases), or a mix of genetic and environmental factors. Examination of this issue as it affects girls is useful. Many females in Canada experience menarche before they leave elementary school. Attaining this milestone does not mean that these females are physically, cognitively, psychologically, or socially "ready" to deal with sexual and reproductive issues. It does mean that families and society must be willing to address the issues, respond in developmentally appropriate ways, and ensure that suitable protection and competent reproductive health care is available.

The AHS data show that adolescents, especially females, who feel that they look older than their age are at considerably greater risk for physical and emotional problems. Compared to other girls their age, they are more likely to have experienced early sexual debut, sexual harassment, and abuse and to use substances such as tobacco and marijuana (Table 7.3).

Table 7.3
Risk factors among British Columbia females who think they look younger than, same age as, and older than same-age peers

	Younger (%)	Same age (%)	Older (%)
Sexual debut at 14 years and younger	6	7	17
Sexually harassed (physically)			
3 or more times in past year	9	8	18
Sexual abuse	14	11	21
Current smoker	12	12	26
Marijuana use in past month	14	16	26

Source: McCreary Centre Society. 1999. BC Adolescent Health Survey, 1998–99. Burnaby, BC: McCreary Centre Society. [Table is original and generated by the present authors.]

SEXUAL DEBUT

As puberty approaches, adolescents experience a heightened aware-ness of the issues of gender, sexual identity, sexual behaviour, and risky behaviours among their peers. Prevailing attitudes among their families, schools, peers, and communities clearly influence this expe-rience. Udry (1990) has investigated the time gap between menarche (female puberty) and age of sexual debut in the United States and notes that the duration of this gap is largely determined by cultural and social factors. In exploring sexual decision making by urban adolescent females in the United States, Paradise et al. (2001, 404) noted that both virginal and sexually experienced girls "view their sexual behavior as being based on personal (although infrequently religious) values." This implies that personal, family, and community values are more influential in shaping the sexual behaviours and lifestyle choices of adolescents than is religion.

The AHS data suggest that there are three distinct sub-groups of adolescents in relation to sexual debut: those who report that they became sexually active at age 14 or younger (11%); those whose sexual debut was at age 15 to 19 years (12%); and the majority of adolescents (77%) who choose to delay engaging in sexual inter-course (McCreary Centre Society 1999a). Early age of sexual initia-tion among adolescents is strongly associated with engagement in unsafe sex practices (Table 7.4). Tobacco and drug use, experience of sexual coercion, and looking older than same-age peers are sig-nificant correlates of early sexual debut among British Columbia students (Table 7.5). As well, the literature identifies ethnicity,

Table 7.4
Sexual debut and unsafe sexual practices among
British Columbia students in grades 7–12

	Sexual debut at 14 years and younger (%)	Sexual debut at 15 years and older (%)
Condom not used last time	43	42
Birth control not used last time*	31	21
Multiple (4 or more) partners in life	35	13
Multiple (2 or more) partners in past 3 months	21	9

* Birth control includes: birth control pills, Depo Provera, diaphragm/contraceptive sponge,
or condom

Source: McCreary Centre Society. 1999. BC Adolescent Health Survey, 1998–99. Burnaby, BC:
McCreary Centre Society. [Table is original and generated by the present authors.]

Table 7.5
Correlates of early sexual debut among British Columbia students in grades 7–12

	Sexual debut at 14 years or or younger	Sexual debut at 15 years and older	Have not had sexual intercourse
Look older than same age peers	47	35	25
Forced/coerced to have sex	20	9	< 1
Used tobacco before age 11	28	11	6
Used alcohol before age 11	32	13	10
Used marijuana before age 11	13	2	1

Source: McCreary Centre Society. 1999. BC Adolescent Health Survey, 1998–99. Burnaby, BC:
McCreary Centre Society. [Table is original and generated by the present authors.]

poverty, experience of abuse, dysfunctional family background, and substance abuse as powerful determinants of early sexual debut (Magnusson 2001; Tapert et al. 2001; Godin and Michaud 1998).

Recent advances in the knowledge base of sexual and reproductive health have implications for early sexual activity. For example, the risk of cervical cancer in adult females is increased by the presence of infection with human papillomavirus (Franco, Duarte-Franco, and Ferenczy 2001). Furthermore, the cervix of the early adolescent is not yet physiologically ready to adequately counteract exposure to HPV (Kahn et al. 2001). This biologic fact, coupled with the tendency of some young adolescents to engage in unsafe sex and experience the equivalent of serial monogamy (i.e., have a sequence of partners), is thought to increase the risk for this form of cancer in young adult females.

That most youth will, sooner or later, become sexually active is not questioned. In an ideal world, the decision to become sexually active would be a matter of individual choice and occur at a time of biopsychosocial readiness. While this decision is clearly an individual matter, common sense suggests that there is such a thing as "too early" a sexual debut. It remains a subject of debate as to what defines "too early" and what, if anything, needs to be done about it. The literature on adolescent sexual and reproductive health is extensive and provides important knowledge about the developmental contexts, behaviours and risks, health promotion and disease prevention options, treatment methodologies, and trends in mortality and morbidity. This literature is of special relevance to policy, programs, and legislation regarding early adolescent sexual debut, but it is often not addressed.

EXPLOITATION AND EARLY DEBUT

Many factors influence when and why an adolescent decides to become sexually active. For some, however, it is not a matter of choice, and their sexual debut results directly from sexual abuse or from a coercive relationship. For others, there are a number of vulnerabilities that may be exploited. Examples include the practice of Internet "lurking," the befriending/predatory practices of pedophiles, and the distribution of "kiddy porn." Such seductive and inappropriate behaviours by older adolescents or adults often result in the introduction of adolescents into drug culture, gang activities, school absenteeism, and involvement in street life. The presence of these indirect risk factors, along with the absence of a caring and supportive parent or adult, is usually associated with early sexual debut.

A contemporary overview of the subject is provided by Bagley and Thurston (1998) and Wolfe (1998) in their chapters in *Determinants of Health: Children and Youth*. A variety of situations can place adolescents at risk for sexual abuse. These include prior physical abuse, dysfunctional family life, school failure, substance abuse, a chronic health condition, being Aboriginal, or being in government care (foster or custodial) (Caputo and Kelly 1998). Sexual abuse can further compromise adolescents' sexual and reproductive health by fostering negative behaviours, such as running away, living on the streets, unsafe sex practices, and alcohol and substance abuse.

Many adolescent females report experiencing sexual harassment and coercive sex. The AHS data indicate that, among girls over 15 years of age, 69% report sexual harassment at school in the previous year, 8% report coercive sex, and 20% report experience of sexual abuse (McCreary Centre Society 1999a). These negative experiences have an impact well beyond the victims' sexual and reproductive health. Adolescents who have been sexually victimized experience higher emotional distress, have lower self-esteem, and may become trapped in self-destructive or risky behaviour patterns. They may also become fearful of disclosure and reticent to seek out mental health or reproductive health services.

Adolescents living on the streets are particularly vulnerable to abuse and exploitation. The profile of street-involved youths in British Columbia's major urban centres (Vancouver and Victoria), however, is quite different from that found in the suburbs or smaller cities. Street youth in larger cities are often older, from outside the area, and less likely to be involved with child protection or educational services (Table 7.6). The city is a much more dangerous milieu for early adolescents; those who become involved in the street scene are immediately at higher risk (McCreary Centre Society 2001a; McCreary Centre Society 1999c).

The literature on violence against youths of both genders is voluminous and we do not reference it. It seems self-evident that having one's personal sexual boundaries violated is hurtful, damages self-esteem, and affects mental health. What may be less evident is that failing to protect children from sexual exploitation or sexual abuse exacts a social toll and leaves each victim with a heavy emotional burden of isolation (sadness), desertion and vulnerability (anger), and self-blame (guilt). This residual emotional damage may be more painful than the sexual assault itself.

POLICY IMPLICATIONS

Adolescent sexuality and reproductive health is not directly addressed in the Convention on the Rights of the Child. Its principles, however, suggest that national governments have responsibilities in three areas, which can be interpreted in terms of the issues of sexuality and reproductive health in adolescence. These include: (a) encouraging legislation defining reproductive rights of all adolescents; (b) advocating for national policies on behalf of accessible, competent,

Table 7.6
Profile of street youth in British Columbia

	Vancouver (n = 145) (%)	Smaller urban centres (n = 284) (%)
Average age	18 years	16 years
Ever in care	44	32
Low family connectedness	97	96
Homeless (no permanent housing)	70	10
Aboriginal	37	27
Not 100% heterosexual	46	26
Currently in school	23	84
Ever expelled or suspended from school	87	84
Sexual abuse	50	40
Ever traded sexual favours	31	23
Sexual debut at 14 years or younger	72	54
Ever been pregnant/caused a pregnancy	33	24

Source: McCreary Centre Society. 1999. BC Street Youth Survey, 2000–01. Burnaby, BC: McCreary Centre Society. [Table is original and generated by the present authors.]

confidential reproductive health care for all adolescents who need it (irrespective of age); and (c) promoting programs focusing on the need for protection from abuse and exploitation of early adolescents. Other responsibilities should include sorting out inconsistencies in application and interpretation of the age of sexual consent and the rights to consent/confidentiality as applied in various child protection, health care, education, research, and juvenile justice systems.

Existing Legislation

Canada has legislation that addresses the adolescent's right to consent to sex. This national statute defines the age (currently 14 years) at which an adolescent can be deemed capable of deciding whether or not to engage in sexual intercourse. The law's intended relevance should not be related to the adolescent's choice – that is, it should not be used to sanction or punish early sexual debut but, rather, to grant police and the courts the legal tools to prosecute pimps and adult offenders. Nonetheless, debates about raising the age of consent to 16 years have become common, but they ignore trends in adolescent behaviour. For example, adolescents are maturing much earlier and 19% of boys and 16% of girls under 17 years are already sexually active, mostly by choice (McCreary Centre Society 1999a).

Given present levels of adolescent sexual activity, it seems inappropriate to change legislation if it renders criminal what is normative adolescent behaviour.

In each province, an Infant's Act spells out the legal age of majority, usually 19 years, and the rights of minors to consent or to refuse medical treatment. While this is an important instrument, it has little direct influence on adolescent behaviour or on most professionals who are called upon to provide treatment. In many agencies, such as hospital emergency rooms and private clinical practices, the front-line reception or nursing staff are not aware of the adolescent's right to consent and to confidentiality. Furthermore, youths in care of the state frequently experience frustration when trying to gain access to medical care and may not know that they have the right to choose their own physician (McCreary Centre Society 1999d).

Health Services and Education

In many countries, national youth health policies place heavy emphasis on sexual and reproductive health. In *A Report from Consultations on a Framework for Sexual and Reproductive Health*, recently authored by Health Canada (1999), however, fewer than one page out of twenty-four addresses youth, and, as a result, the report reflects the tendency to meld youth with adult issues and omit youth-specific input to policy formulation. Many family planning and sexual health services expect adolescents to fit into what are essentially adult-oriented programs. National policies must become more specific about adolescents' service needs, standards of sexual and reproductive health care, and special issues such as those raised by early age of sexual maturity. Within that context, policies need to foster and evaluate health-promoting/disease-preventing strategies that target adolescents at risk for early sexual debut and its attendant concerns.

In a matter of a few decades, the range of effective contraceptive technologies, such as injectable and emergency contraceptives, has expanded enormously. In addition, the introduction of modern antibiotics and access to safe, legalized abortions have changed the outcomes of many STDs and unplanned pregnancies among adolescents. Access to these alternatives becomes a contemporary issue for sexually active teens, although controversy over harm reduction strategies, such as condom dispensers in schools, remains a sensitive topic in schools and communities. The newer problems associated

Table 7.7
STD prevention knowledge among British Columbia students in grades 7–12

	Not at all effective in STD prevention (%)	Somewhat effective in STD prevention (%)	Very effective in STD prevention (%)	Don't know (%)
Condoms	4	39	43	15
Birth control pill	33	26	21	21
Asking partner to be tested	8	25	47	20
Abstinence	6	4	76	14

Source: Natalie Franz and Colleen Poon. *Making Choices: Sex, Ethnicity and BC Youth.* 2000. Burnaby, BC: McCreary Centre Society. [Table is original and generated by the present authors.]

with hepatitis B and C and youths' risk of exposure to HIV/AIDS, especially when coupled with low rates of condom use, have introduced new policy pressures in this regard.

Lack of knowledge about normal adolescent development hampers effective adolescent reproductive health care. Commonly held negative attitudes towards the emerging sexuality of today's adolescents are an important source of resistance to addressing their needs. Adolescents themselves often lack appropriate information about their own development. While the Internet has put pornography at young people's fingertips, it also provides access to many useful web-based, youth-oriented information and chat services about sexual health. The extent to which adolescents use the information available through these sources is unclear. Sixty-four percent of Canadian adolescents report that they have attended sex education classes at school (Statistics Canada 1998). It is uncertain, however, whether this education is translated into actual knowledge. The AHS assessed British Columbia students' knowledge of STD prevention and found that fewer than half (43%) replied that condoms were very effective in STD prevention, and only 33% knew that oral contraceptives did not prevent STDs (Table 7.7). In addition, only 59% of sexually active British Columbia adolescents over 14 years of age used a condom the last time they had sex, and 21% used withdrawal, or no method, to prevent pregnancy the last time they had sexual intercourse (Table 7.8). When asked whom they would go to first for issues related to contraception or STDs, fewer than half of adolescents listed health professionals (Table 7.9). Clearly, there are gaps in young people's knowledge and less than optimal

Table 7.8
Condom and birth control use among sexually active British Columbia students

	14 years and younger (%)	15 years and older (%)
Condom used last time	57	59
Birth control used last time:		
Birth control pill	30	40
Other method	3	2
Withdrawal	9	11
No method	20	10

Source: McCreary Centre Society. 1999. *BC Adolescent Health Survey, 1998–99*. Burnaby, British Columbia: McCreary Centre Society. [Table is original and generated by the present authors.]

Table 7.9
Help-seeking among sexually active British Columbia students in grades 7–12

	14 years and younger (%)	15 years and older (%)
Preferred source of help with needing birth control information:		
Parent	20	16
Peer	12	17
Health professional	28	42
No one/not sure	28	18
Preferred source of help with STDs:		
Parent	23	19
Peer	12	13
Health professional	38	48
No one/not sure	19	14

Source: McCreary Centre Society. 1999. *BC Adolescent Health Survey, 1998–99*. Burnaby, BC: McCreary Centre Society. [Table is original and generated by the present authors.]

likelihood of gaining access to reproductive services, despite Canada's long history of health promotion programs in schools and in the community. Adolescents' life skills, such as refusal skills, proper use of condoms, and help-seeking strategies, seem to need further development and reinforcement.

Early Sexual Debut

Early sexual debut should be a significant social concern. It places young adolescents at risk for sexual exploitation, sexually transmitted diseases and teen pregnancy, risky behaviours, abusive relationships, family conflict, and educational disruption. For this group, however, the needed response is not legislative but programmatic. Here the articles of the Convention on the Rights of the Child that address rights to competent care provided in privacy, respect for confidentiality, and observing the adolescent's right to informed consent are particularly relevant. These principles should be the foundation of any program.

Most health promotion practices and prevention services fail to adequately differentiate between the needs of adolescents based on the age at which they become sexually active and, specifically, the high-risk group of those who debut early. Models and mechanisms for delivering pregnancy control, STD/AIDS treatment, and alcohol and drug abuse services lack integration or coordination to encourage their use by early adolescents. Early adolescents who are sexually active (or contemplating becoming so) have a greater need for reliable, understandable information, clear presentation of options, and easy access to such services as emergency contraception, abortion/adoption counselling, and treatment of STDs. These services must be provided directly to the adolescent, must encourage involvement of sexual partners, and must be sensitive to the continuing role of parents and family during early adolescence.

Neither national policy nor the United Nations Convention (Article 5, evolving capacities of the child) adequately addresses the implications of biologic or psychosocial variability due to early or late maturation. At a program level, sexual or reproductive health needs of special populations, such as youths with chronic illnesses, disabilities, or mental challenge, are commonly ignored. In some jurisdictions, there may be a one- to two-year gap in service coverage between youth and adult health care systems: care is not offered by one sector (because the individual is seen as being too old) and is denied by the other (because he or she is considered too young).

Society's responses to adolescent sexuality are often ambiguous or inappropriate. How do we identify and address the needs of adolescents who choose to engage in early sexual activity within a societal context that favours virginity and promotes abstinence? Are they to be considered normal or deviant? Do we respond by criminalizing their behaviour, denying them needed health services, or penalizing them socially by expelling them from school? Teen pregnancy prevention programs that take a "just say no" approach and similar abstinence promotion programs have, on their own, had little effect on teen pregnancy rates in the United States (Christopher and Roosa 1990). On the other hand, programs that link traditional family values, religious beliefs, or academic expectations create a social context in which strategies such as promoting abstinence can be more effective (Kirby et al. 1994; Paradise et al. 2001). While such programs do not eliminate the ever-present risks of early sexual debut in some adolescents, they may delay exposure in others.

Exploitation and Abuse: Street and Homeless Youth

All Western societies seek to protect their adolescents from sexual exploitation and abuse. Each province in Canada has enacted child protection legislation and introduced a range of provincially man-dated child protection services. At the federal level, the Criminal Code addresses various aspects of this issue and pays special atten-tion to offenders. Unfortunately, in neither of these jurisdictions has legislation proven itself sufficient in the battle against the sexual exploitation and sexual abuse of adolescents. At the international level, some agreements stemming from the Convention on the Rights of the Child have recently prompted domestic legislation for the protection of children; for example, the Optional Protocol to the Rights of the Child on the Sale of Children, Child Prostitution, and Child Pornography (United Nations 2000).

Canada continues to be uncertain about the definition of sexual abuse and the boundaries that child protection services should observe. Jurisdictions also vary in the extent to which their services give priority to younger children or to youths over 15 years of age. Many programs are less flexible when dealing with non-compliant youths or those with multiple problems. Youths in conflict with the law and families in chaos receive varying levels of child protec-tion services. Professional groups, such as physicians, and even ordinary citizens, are required, by law, to report suspected sexual abuse, but many are reluctant to do so. While some safeguards and services are in place, the degree to which they address the needs of sexually exploited or abused adolescents is unknown. AHS data report a decrease in sexual abuse of females in British Columbia from 21% in 1992 to 15% in 1998 (McCreary Centre Society 1999b). While this is encouraging news, the number of affected individuals still potentially amounts to a provincial caseload of thirty thousand adolescents.

The data suggest that the mere existence of provincial child protection statutes is not enough: an urgent need exists for more accurate information on the true incidence of sexual abuse and exploitation of adolescents. It is not enough to depend only on reported cases. Despite aggressive public information strategies, such as school-based prevention programs and anonymous reporting opportunities (crisis lines, agency confidentiality), abuse continues to be significantly underreported. British Columbia's Children's Commissioner and the Advocate for Children and Youth independently report that provincial child protection services struggle with human resource shortfalls that compromise follow-up and case management. These deficiencies can mean that the abused adolescent is also victimized by the system. A recent study of street-involved youths in British Columbia showed that 69% are, or have been, involved with child welfare or youth justice services; most (57%) are still living at home or in care and most (62%) still have some connection with school (McCreary Centre Society 2001a). It would seem reasonable to ask: are the adolescents failing to use the services? or are the services failing to reach the adolescents?

With regard to street youth, a number of provinces have already introduced legislation allowing agencies to place high-risk young adolescents living on the street in short-term secure care. While well intentioned, this legislation will not be effective unless matched by adequately resourced programs and conducted in accordance with accepted principles of youth-friendly care. It seems reasonable, given the British Columbia experience, to place more emphasis and resources upstream, before adolescents reach the streets of large urban areas.

In reviewing the issues of street and homeless youth in Canada, Caputo and Kelly (1998) report that the priority needs of youth are related to drug use and safe housing, not to sexual and reproductive health. Their findings are in keeping with those from British Columbia. In the context of the sexual and reproductive health needs of high-risk adolescents, provincial legislation and provincial youth policy that targets adolescent sexual behaviours will likely be less effective than targeted, locally based, comprehensive early intervention programs that address identified needs.

YOUTH-POSITIVE SOCIETY

The concept of "youth" is recent, socially driven, and culturally defined (Levi and Schmitt 1997). Only recently has adolescence become the subject of systematic study. Currently, this period of development is receiving new recognition, and the contribution of the health sector to adolescent development has become a topic of renewed interest (Federal, Provincial, and Territorial Advisory Committee on Population Health 2000). Central to these discussions is an acknowledgment of adolescent sexuality and the challenges of promoting reproductive health through greater emphasis on resilience and on youth participation (Langille et al. 1998; Pan American Health Organization 1998; Tonkin 1997; United Nations Secretariat 1999).

There is growing agreement that healthy adolescent development is maximized in the context of a youth-positive society (Burt 1998; Pan American Health Organization 1998; Tonkin 1997; United Nations Secretariat 1999). A youth-positive society is one that values adolescents for who they are; it embraces the principles and articles of the Convention on the Rights of the Child, especially those that relate to meaningful youth participation and youth empowerment. A youth-positive society is one that ensures that youth issues are on the agenda at the family, school, community, provincial, national, and global levels. Unfortunately, as United Nations, UNICEF, and International Planned Parenthood Federation documents attest, a global agenda for youth remains a distant future goal.

Achievement of a youth-positive society in Canada would be facilitated by a national youth policy and a national youth health agenda. Such steps should be preceded, however, by greater efforts to ensure that the voices of youths are heard at every level and that their meaningful participation in setting youth-related agendas is properly supported. There are a growing number of examples of how youth participation has been practised in British Columbia, such as McCreary's B4 and Next Steps projects (Ward 2005; Sadler, Murphy, and McCreary Centre Society 2006), and elsewhere in Canada, such as the Centre of Excellence for Youth Engagement (http://www.tgmag.ca/centres/). Another approach is the application at the adolescent level of the "assets framework" developed by the Search Institute in Minneapolis (http://www.search-institute.org/). Canada must learn from these models and make a serious commitment to policies that enhance the user-friendliness of existing sexual and reproductive health services for youth. For example, recommendations of youths themselves for youth sex education include the use of peer educators, provision of sex education to younger youths and "refresher" classes for older youths, as well as information focused on STD and pregnancy prevention rather than on the "mechanics" of sex (McCreary Centre Society 2001b.). There is no guarantee that the development of accessible, comprehensive "one-stop shops" for youth health and social services, or of youth-specific programs within existing services, will promote sexual and reproductive health among mainstream adolescents; these adolescents are more likely to turn to friends, family, or traditional family practice and family planning clinics. Such programs would, however, be helpful in reaching high-risk, marginalized youths, including those who are street-involved, homeless, Aboriginal, gay-lesbian-bisexual-transgender-questioning, chronically ill, or out of school. Services for high-risk youths may also need to broaden their scope to address other primary concerns of youths, such as safe emergency housing, affordable longer-term housing, vocational and educational supports, and alcohol and addiction treatment. Such services, if comprehensive, would include access to sexual and reproductive health care.

CONCLUSION

We are all sexual beings. Our children must pass safely through adolescence and its attendant risks, including those related to sexuality. The role of legislation is limited. It should protect the rights of adolescents and ensure them as safe a passage as possible in their transition to adulthood. Policies that embrace the spirit as well as the letter of the United Nations Convention on the Rights of the Child are long overdue. National policies can have a broad reach by advocating for youth and promoting youth-positive development.

There is a growing recognition of the need for a significant shift in adolescent policy frameworks and program strategies. The Government of New Zealand's document *Youth Development Strategy Aotearoa* provides an example of such a shift (Ministry of Youth Affairs 2002). Researchers in Minnesota, Melbourne, Gothenburg, Vancouver, and Boston are developing the evidence base in favour of policies and practices for youth-positive development, which involves moving away from perceiving youths as the "problem" towards acknowledging youths as part of the "solution." Such policies are being advocated by the Pan American Health Organization, UNICEF, and foundations such as the W.T. Grant Foundation. They have as their goal the promotion of resiliency and connectedness, reinforcing the importance of families, peers, and schools in setting a positive tone and emphasizing a youth's assets and the creation of youth-friendly health services. As well, there continues to be a need for competent, caring, comprehensive services that enable young people to connect (and reconnect) with their families and that offer them the experience of continuity of relationships with caring adults. Finally, a youth-positive society would offer a different "vocabulary" when discussing youths and their issues.

The way that adults address the sexual and reproductive health of adolescents is analogous to the position of these young people in contemporary society. To influence sexual behaviour and to promote safe sex practices among today's youth, we must change some of our own attitudes and practices. This change of perspective requires us to address adolescent issues and needs by helping them to value themselves, their health, and their connections with others. This change also requires us to reconsider the significance of early sexual debut, to be more creative and protective in the face of exploitation and sexual abuse, and to understand what it is that sexually active adolescents seek when they approach us for care. If we can grasp those opportunities, we will learn more about adolescents as persons. Only then can we begin to help them see their issues less as problems and more as a part of the process of becoming fully functioning adults.

NOTES

1 In Chapter 2 of this book, the author points to Article 5, which mentions the rights of parents but in conjunction with the nebulous concept of evolving capacities as follows: "Article 5 recognizes the rights and duties of parents to provide appropriate direction and guidance to the child, when he or she is exercising rights, 'in a manner consistent with the evolving capacities of the child.'"

2 The AHS data reported as percentages in the text and tables may vary according to the particular denominator upon which they are based. While standard deviations and statistical tests of significance have not been applied to these data, our statistical consultants advise that there are no significant design effects and that – given the large sample size and

the high response rate – this random sample produced differences in reported frequencies that are significant. In Table 7.6, a small convenience sample was used and reported differences are not necessarily significant. For further information on the AHS methodology, the reader is referred to www.mcs.bc.ca.

REFERENCES

Adolescent Medicine: Challenge of the 1990's. 1991. 8th Canadian Ross Conference in Paediatrics. Ottawa: Canadian Paediatric Society.

Alan Guttmacher Institute. 1998. *Into a New World: Young Women's Sexual and Reproductive Lives.* New York: Alan Guttmacher Institute.

Annie E. Casey Foundation. 1998. *When Teens Have Sex: Issues and Trends.* A "Kids Count" Special Report. Baltimore: Annie E. Casey Foundation.

Bagley, Christopher, and Wilfreda E. Thurston. 1998. Decreasing child sexual abuse. In *Canada Health Action: Building on the Legacy. Papers Commissioned by the National Forum on Health.* Vol. 1: *Determinants of Health: Children and Youth*, 133–73. Sainte Foy, QC: Éditions MultiMondes.

Barker, G. 2000. *What about boys? A Literature Review on the Health and Development of Adolescent Boys.* Geneva: World Health Organization.

Bibby, Reginald W. 2001. *Canada's Teens: Today, Yesterday, and Tomorrow.* Toronto: Stoddart.

Boyce, W.F., M. Doherty, D. MacKinnon, and C. Fortin. 2003. *Canadian Youth, Sexual Health and HIV/AIDS Study.* Toronto: Council of Ministers of Education (Canada).

British Columbia Provincial Health Officer. 1996. *A Report on the Health of British Columbians: Provincial Health Officer's Annual Report 1995.* Victoria, BC: Ministry of Health and Ministry Responsible for Seniors.

Burt, M.R. 1998. *Why Should We Invest in Adolescence?* Washington, DC: PAHO.

Caputo, Tullio, and Katherine Kelly. 1998. Improving the health of street/homeless youth. In *Canada Health Action: Building on the Legacy. Papers Commissioned by the National Forum on Health. Volume 1: Determinants of Health: Children and Youth*, 408–40. Sainte Foy, QC: Éditions MultiMondes.

Centers for Disease Control and Prevention (United States). 2001. *Fact Sheet: Youth Risk Behavior Trends*. www.cdc.gov/nccdphp/dash/yrbs/trend.htm. Retrieved 1 August 2006.

Christopher, S.F., and M. Roosa. 1990. An evaluation of an adolescent pregnancy prevention program: Is "Just say no" enough? *Family Relations* 39:68–72.

Currie, C., Samdal, O., Boyce, W., and Smith, B. 2001. *Health Behaviour in School-aged Children: A World Health Organization Cross-National Study*. Research Protocol for the 2001/02 Survey. Edinburgh, Scotland: University of Edinburgh, Child and Adolescent Health Research Unit.

Federal, Provincial, and Territorial Advisory Committee on Population Health. 2000. *The Opportunity of Adolescence: The Health Sector Contribution*. Ottawa: Minister of Public Works and Government Services.

Franco, E.L., E. Duarte-Franco, and A. Ferenczy. 2001. Cervical cancer: Epidemiology, prevention, and the role of human papillomavirus infection. *Canadian Medical Association Journal* 164(7):1017–25.

Godin, Gaston, and Francine Michaud. 1998. STD and AIDS prevention among young people. In *Canada Health Action: Building on the Legacy. Papers Commissioned by the National Forum on Health*. Vol. 1: *Determinants of Health: Children and Youth*, 357–400. Sainte-Foy, QC: Éditions MultiMondes.

Haffner, D., ed. 1995. *Facing Facts: Sexual Health for America's Adolescents*. The Report of the National Commission on Adolescent Sexual Health. New York: Sexuality Information and Education Council of the United States.

Health Canada. 1999. *A Report from Consultations on a Framework for Sexual and Reproductive Health*. Ottawa: Health Canada.

Kahn, Jessica A., Susan L. Rosenthal, Paul A. Succop, Gloria Y.F. Ho, and Robert D. Burk. 2001. *Mediators of the Association between Coitarche and HPV Acquisition*. Annual Meeting of the Society for Adolescent Medicine, March. San Diego, CA: Society for Adolescent Medicine.

Kaltiala-Heino, Riittakerttu, Matti Rimpelä, Aila Rissanen, and Päivi Rantanen. 2001. Early puberty and early sexual activity are associated with bulimic-type eating pathology in middle adolescence. *Journal of Adolescent Medicine* 28:346–52.

Kidder, K., J. Stein, and J. Fraser. 2000. *The Health of Canada's Children: A CICH Profile*. 3rd ed. Ottawa: Canadian Institute of Child Health (CICH).

King, Alan J.C., R.P. Beazley, W.K. Warren, C.A. Hankins, A.S. Robertson, and J.L. Radford. 1988. *Canada Youth and AIDS Study.* Kingston, ON: Social Program Evaluation Group, Queen's University.

King, Alan J.C., William F. Boyce, and Matthew A. King. 1999. *Trends in the Health of Canadian Youth.* Ottawa: Health Canada.

Kirby, D., L. Short, J. Collins, D. Rugg, L. Kolbe, M. Howard, B. Miller, R. Sonenstein, and L.S. Zabin. 1994. School-based programs to reduce sexual risk behaviors: A review of effectiveness. *Public Health Reports* 109(3):339–59.

Langille, D.B., P. Andreou, R.P. Beazley, and M.E. Delaney. 1998. Sexual health knowledge of students at a high school in Nova Scotia. *Canadian Journal of Public Health* 89(2):85–9.

Levi, Giovanni, and Jean-Claude Schmitt, eds. 1997. *A History of Young People in the West. Volume 2: Stormy Evolution to Modern Times,* trans. Carol Volk. Cambridge: Belknap Press of Harvard University Press.

Magnusson, Chris. 2001. Adolescent girls' sexual attitudes and opposite-sex relations in 1970 and in 1996. *Journal of Adolescent Health* 28:242–52.

McCreary Centre Society. 1999a. *BC Adolescent Health Survey (1998–99).* Burnaby, BC: McCreary Centre Society.

– 1999b. *Healthy Connections: Listening to BC Youth. Highlights from the Adolescent Health Survey II.* Burnaby, BC: McCreary Centre Society.

– 1999c. *Our Kids Too: Sexually Exploited Youth in British Columbia. An Adolescent Health Survey.* Burnaby, BC: McCreary Centre Society.

– 1999d. *The Doctor Project ... for Healthier Youth in Care.* Burnaby, BC: McCreary Centre Society.

– 2001a. *No Place to Call Home: A Profile of Street Youth in British Columbia.* Burnaby, BC: McCreary Centre Society.

– 2001b. *Our Communities – Our Health: Young People Discuss Solutions to Their Health Issues.* Burnaby, BC: McCreary Centre Society.

Ministry of Youth Affairs. 2002. *Youth Development Strategy Aotearoa.* Wellington, New Zealand: Ministry of Youth Affairs. http://www.myd.govt.nz/uploads/docs/0.7.6.5%20ydsa.pdf. Retrieved 28 July 2006.

Pan American Health Organization (PAHO). 1998. *Plan of Action for Health and Development of Adolescents and Youth in the Americas 1998–2001.* Washington, DC: PAHO.

Paradise, Jan E., Jennifer Cote, Sara Minsky, Ana Lourenco, and Jonathan Howland. 2001. Personal values and sexual decision-making

among virginal and sexually experienced urban adolescent girls.
Journal of Adolescent Health 28:404–9.

Patrick, D.M., T. Wong, and R.A. Jordan. 2000. Sexually transmitted
infections in Canada: Recent resurgence threatens national goals.
Canadian Journal of Human Sexuality 9:149–65.

Rodriguez-Garcia, R., J.S. Russell, M. Maddaleno, and M. Kastrinakis.
2000. *The Legislative and Policy Environment for Adolescent Health
in Latin America and the Caribbean.* Washington, DC: PAHO.

Rutter, Michael. 1979. *Changing Youth in a Changing Society: Patterns
of Adolescent Development and Disorder.* London: Nuffield Provincial
Hospitals Trust.

Sadler, D., Murphy, A., and McCreary Centre Society. 2006. *The Next
Steps: BC Youths' Response to the* AHS *III and Ideas for Action.*
A project of the Adolescent Health Survey III. Vancouver, BC:
McCreary Centre Society.

Senderowitz, Judith. 1997. *Reproductive Health Outreach Programs for
Young Adults.* Washington: Pathfinder International.

Statistics Canada. 1998. *Survey of Consumer Finances 1998: Individuals,
Aged 15 Years and Over, with and without Income, 1997 Income.*
Public-use microdata file. Ottawa: Statistics Canada. [Results of the
National Population Health Survey, Cycle 2, 1996/97.]

Tanner, J.M. 1978. *Fetus into Man: Physical Growth from Conception to
Maturity.* Cambridge: Harvard University Press.

Tapert, Susan F., Gregory A. Aarons, Georganna R. Sedlar, and Sandra
A. Brown. 2001. Adolescent substance use and sexual risk-taking
behavior. *Journal of Adolescent Health* 28:181–9.

Thomas, B. Helen, Alba DiCenso, and Lauren Griffith. 1998a.
Adolescent sexual behaviour: Results from an Ontario sample. Part I:
Adolescent sexual activity. *Canadian Journal of Public Health*
89(2):90–3.

– 1998b. Adolescent sexual behaviour: Results from an Ontario sample.
Part II: Use of protection. *Canadian Journal of Public Health*
89(2):94–7.

Tolman, Deborah L. 1999. Femininity as a barrier to positive sexual
health for adolescent girls. *Journal of the American Medical Women's
Association* 54:133–8.

Tonkin, Roger S. 1997. The future needs of Canada's youth. In *Child
and Youth Health Care in the 21st Century,* 93–100. 11th Canadian
Ross Conference in Paediatrics. Ottawa: Canadian Paediatric Society.

- 2001a. A view from the trenches: Perspectives on population-based adolescent health research. *International Journal of Adolescent Medicine and Health* 13(1):45–51.
- 2001b. Youth and the National Children's Agenda. *Journal of Paediatrics and Child Health* 6(4):1–2.
- In press. Early intervention: With an adolescent twist. *Journal of Paediatrics and Child Health.*
Udry, J. Richard. 1990. Hormonal and social determinants of adolescent sexual initiation. In *Kinsey Institute Series.* Vol. 3: *Adolescence and Puberty*, ed. John Bancroft and June Machover, 70–8. New York: Oxford University Press.
United Nations. 1989. *Convention on the Rights of the Child.* Geneva: United Nations.
- 2000. *Optional Protocol to the Convention on the Rights of the Child on the Sale of Children, Child Prostitution and Child Pornography.* Geneva: United Nations. http://www.unhchr.ch/html/menu2/ dopchild.htm. Retrieved 1 August 2006.
United Nations Secretariat. 1999. *Youth Information Bulletin,* vols. 1–2, nos. 98–9. New York: United Nations Secretariat.
Ward, Laura. 2005. 9th Annual B4: Breaking Barriers and Building Bridges. McCreary Centre Society, Vancouver, BC, 18–20 March.
Wolfe, David A. 1998. Prevention of child abuse and neglect. In *Canada Health Action: Building on the Legacy. Papers Commissioned by the National Forum on Health.* Vol. 1: *Determinants of Health: Children and Youth*, 104–131. Sainte Foy, QC: Éditions MultiMondes.
World Health Organization (WHO). 1985. *Reproductive Health in Adolescence: Position Paper.* Geneva: WHO.

8

Substance Use: Harm Reduction and the Rights of the Canadian Adolescent

CHRISTIANE POULIN

Harm reduction is increasingly contemplated as an alternative philosophy and strategy to the dominant paradigm of primary prevention regarding substance use by adolescent populations. Adolescence is a life stage characterized by increasing autonomy. The wide variability in emotional, social, and intellectual development during this life stage, however, gives rise to uncertainty and/or disagreement about adolescents' decision-making capacity both in general and concerning illegal behaviours such as substance use. Some adolescents may have neither the confidence nor the skills to achieve full autonomy, despite their need to free themselves from the authority of adults (Ames and Miller 1994).

Proponents of a harm reduction approach focus on the inevitability of substance use at the population level. They also focus on pragmatic ways in which the consequences of use can be mitigated for the drug user and the community. For many persons, however, the problem with harm reduction is that, by not actively condemning drug use, it seems to passively condone it. For proponents of a legal approach to drug use, any use of drugs is viewed as essentially undesirable, whether or not it results in harmful consequences. By contrast, harm reduction advocates suggest consideration of the complex interplay between the physiologic effects of a specific drug, the attributes of the person using the drug, and the manner and context in which the drug is used in order to arrive at an understanding of the real harm arising from drug use and the ways in which such harm can be minimized.

The past twenty-five years have seen an increasing acceptance of harm reduction as a goal and a strategy for addressing substance use in Canada and in several other countries. The purpose of this chapter is to interpret harm reduction as it pertains to Canadian adolescents, using the United Nations Convention on the Rights of the Child as a policy framework. With reference to articles from the Convention considered salient in the debate on harm reduction, this chapter discusses whether harm reduction is a reasonable stance and how it might be implemented for both mainstream and street-involved adolescents relative to their use of alcohol, tobacco, cannabis, and other substances.

TWO FRAMEWORKS FOR CONTROLLING ADOLESCENT SUBSTANCE USE

Canada's Drug Strategy

Adolescence is a life stage during which decisions and choices about alcohol and other substance use are often first made. A high percentage of adolescents use one or more substances in the course of a year. For example, in a sample of 13,549 adolescent students (average age of 15.2 years) from Canada's four Atlantic provinces, more than 57% reported having used at least one substance in 1998, the most commonly used substances being alcohol, tobacco, and cannabis (Barcelo, Jones, and Grobe 1998; MacDonald and Holmes 1998; Poulin and Baker 1998; Van Til, MacMillan, and Poulin 1998).

For Canadian adolescents, these substances are illegal either through provincial laws prohibiting the sale of such substances to persons under a specified age or through a federal Act specifying the criminal offences associated with using illicit substances. Clearly, the goal of such legislation is abstinence, at least until the attainment of the legal age, in the case of alcohol and tobacco, and throughout the entire lifespan, in the case of illicit substances.

Canada's official stance, however, outside the legal system, is that "[b]ecause substance abuse is primarily a health issue rather than an enforcement issue, harm reduction is considered to be a realistic, pragmatic, and humane approach as opposed to attempting solely to reduce the use of drugs" (Health Canada 1998, 4). Canada's response to the problem of substance abuse, as articulated in Canada's Drug Strategy from 1992 to 1997 and reaffirmed in 1998, is therefore "to reduce the harm associated with alcohol and other drugs to individuals, families and communities" (ibid.).

Three of the five objectives of Canada's Drug Strategy speak directly to youth-related issues. The first objective is to "reduce the demand for drugs," particularly illicit drugs among youths, with emphasis on "hard drugs" such as cocaine, LSD, speed, and heroin. The second objective is to "reduce drug-related mortality and morbidity," with mention made of high-risk patterns of alcohol and other drug use. The third objective is to "improve the effectiveness of and accessibility to substance abuse information and interventions" by identifying and promoting best practices in substance abuse prevention, education, treatment, and rehabilitation.

Thus, harm reduction as a goal and a strategy to address adolescent substance use appears to be supported by Canada's Drug Strategy. In practice, however, there is little understanding or consensus about what exactly is meant by harm reduction as it pertains to the adolescent population.

In the case of adult drug users, there is a clear acceptance of the user's autonomy in making decisions about substance use and participation in interventions to reduce harm. In the case of persons involved in illicit substance use, such as cocaine or heroin, the goals and means of harm reduction can be articulated explicitly. In the case of underage street youth, involvement in substance use brings such a high risk of serious harm to those who have already identified themselves as autonomous that the pragmatic stance of harm reduction is acceptable to agencies that provide support and services. The major debate around harm reduction as pertains to adolescents, therefore, centres around underage youths still in school and/or living at home and involved in either licit or illicit substance use.

United Nations Convention on the Rights of the Child

The 1989 United Nations Convention on the Rights of the Child, ratified by Canada in 1991, identifies civil, political, economic, social, and cultural rights of the child related to survival, development, protection, and participation (the definition of child being inclusive of those aged 18 and under) (United Nations 1989). The Convention recognizes public order and morals and duties of the state with regard to the rights of the adolescent. It stresses in many articles the notion of the adolescent's rights being in accordance with age, maturity, and evolving capacity, and it also recognizes limitations to the adolescent's rights as prescribed by law. Thus, the Convention provides the basis for balancing public good versus individual freedom for a segment of the population not emancipated by virtue of age. The inclusion of rights, duties, and limitations makes the Convention a valuable framework to inform the debate on harm reduction strategies for adolescents.

VIEWS ON HARM REDUCTION
IN THE TWO FRAMEWORKS

Use of Illicit Substances

There is no generally accepted definition of the term "harm reduction" (Riley et al. 1999). According to Marlatt, Somers, and Tapert (1993), harm reduction focuses on the impact of addictive behaviour instead of drug use itself. It takes the position that elimination of risky behaviours such as illicit drug use is unrealistic. The wide range of policies considered to be part of a harm reduction approach are designed to minimize the negative consequences of addiction and are evaluated in terms of their benefit to the individual drug user and to the greater society.

A key part of the debate on harm reduction centres on the role of abstinence. Clearly, abstinence can be a means of effecting a decrease in harmful effects experienced by individuals and communities. For strong proponents of harm reduction, however, only those policies and programs that specifically aim to reduce drug-related harm, without requiring abstinence, fall under the rubric of harm reduction.

With regard to the United Nations Convention, Article 33 stipulates that "States Parties shall take all appropriate measures, including legislative, administrative, social and educational measures, to protect children from the illicit use of narcotic drugs and psychotropic substances as defined in the relevant international treaties, and to prevent the use of children in the illicit production and trafficking of such substances" (United Nations 1989).

Article 33 therefore proposes abstinence as the sole goal of measures to protect children from psychotropic substances. Similarly, the first objective of Canada's Drug Strategy speaks to demand reduction, rather than to harm reduction, in the case of youth use of illicit drugs such as cocaine, LSD, speed, and heroin. Thus, Article 33 and Canada's Drug Strategy appear to agree on a goal of

Table 8.1
Estimated past-year prevalence of substance use by adolescent students
(12–19 years old) in Canadian Provinces

Province	Alcohol (%)	Tobacco (%)	Cannabis (%)
Newfoundland & Labrador[1]	58.3	38.1	30.2
Nova Scotia[2]	56.7	36.1	37.7
New Brunswick[3]	55.7	32.6	30.9
Prince Edward Island[4]	52.5	26.5	21.7
Ontario[5]	65.7	28.3	29.2
Manitoba[6]	80.4	39.5	37.9

Sources:
[1] MacDonald, C.A., and P.R. Holmes. 1998. *Newfoundland and Labrador Student Drug Use 1998. Technical Report.* St John's: Government of Newfoundland and Labrador, Department of Health, Addictions Services.
[2] Poulin, C., and J. Baker. 1998. *Nova Scotia Student Drug Use 1998. Technical Report.* Halifax: Nova Scotia Department of Health and Dalhousie University.
[3] Barcelo, A., B. Jones, and C. Grobe. 1998. *Provincial Student Drug Use Survey. Highlights 1998.* Fredericton: New Brunswick Department of Health and Community Services, Provincial Epidemiology Service.
[4] Van Til, L., H. MacMillan, and C. Poulin. 1998. *Prince Edward Island Student Drug Use 1998. Technical Report.* Charlottetown: Prince Edward Island, Department of Health and Social Services.
[5] Adlaf, E.M., A. Paglia, F.J. Ivis, and A. Ialomiteanu. 2000. Nonmedical drug use among adolescent students: Highlights from the 1999 Ontario Student Drug Use Survey. *Canadian Medical Association Journal* 162(12):1677–1680.
[6] Patton, D., D. Brown, B. Broszeit, and J. Dhaliwal. 2001. *Substance Use among Manitoba High School Students.* Winnipeg: Addictions Foundation of Manitoba. http://www.afm.mb.ca/Research/documents/HSSU.pdf. Retrieved 1 August 2007.

abstinence in the case of hard drugs. The main inconsistency between Article 33 and Canada's Drug Strategy pertains to cannabis use.

Cannabis is the illicit substance most commonly used by adolescents in many countries, including Canada (Table 8.1), the United States, and Europe. In 1998, the estimated annual prevalence of cannabis use among adolescent students in the Atlantic provinces ranged from 22% in Prince Edward Island to 38% in Nova Scotia (Barcelo, Jones, and Grobe 1998; MacDonald and Holmes 1998; Poulin and Baker 1998; Van Til, MacMillan, and Poulin 1998). In 1999, 30% of students in Ontario reported cannabis use, while an estimated 38% of students in Manitoba used cannabis in 2001 (Adlaf et al. 2000; Patton et al. 2001). By contrast, the estimated annual prevalence of cocaine or heroin use among adolescent students in those six provinces ranged from 2% to 4%.

Cannabis is used in a wide array of contexts with greater or lesser risk of harm. The main acute adverse health effects of cannabis include anxiety and panic reactions as well as motor vehicle accidents due to an amplification of impairment caused by a concurrent use of alcohol (Hall and Solowij 1998). Chronic heavy cannabis use has been shown to be associated with diverse negative health consequences, such as chronic bronchitis, cannabis dependence syndrome, subtle impairments of attention and memory, and adverse effects on reproduction (Hall and Solowij 1998). The health risks of cannabis use are far less grave than are those associated with cocaine or heroin use. Of the estimated 805 deaths related to illicit drug use that occurred in Canada in 1995, opiate and cocaine poisoning accounted for about 20% and 10%, respectively (Single et al. 2000). By contrast, while cannabis has sometimes been detected in the toxicologic profiles of drug overdose cases investigated by medical examiners or coroners in Canada, such deaths are rarely attributed to cannabis (Poulin, Stein, and Butt 1998; Poulin 1997). According to Hall and Solowij (1998), there are no confirmed, published cases worldwide of human deaths from cannabis poisoning.

Based on the above health risks and the high prevalence of use, there is justification for considering harm reduction strategies in the case of cannabis use by adolescents in Canada. Certainly, Canada's Drug Strategy seems to allow for a distinction between hard drugs and cannabis as used by adolescents. In contrast, Article 33 of the Convention, as mentioned earlier, does not differentiate between the various psychotropic substances that fall under international treaties, except for narcotics. The lack of differentiation between use and abuse, and among substances according to their context of use, harms, and risks, represents a limitation of Article 33. Thus, the Convention and Canada's Drug Strategy differ in their stance: the former is inflexible as to the substance, while the latter recognizes the epidemiology and risk of adolescent substance use.

Adolescents' Increasing Autonomy

Articles 5, 12, and 13 of the Convention make explicit the relevance of the child's age, maturity, and evolving capacity to the issue of adolescent rights within the context of parental responsibility, community involvement and local custom, and legal constraints. These articles provide a rational basis for debating harm reduction as the potential philosophical underpinning of substance use interventions that take account of adolescents' increasing autonomy.

Article 5 reads: "States Parties shall respect the responsibilities, rights and duties of parents or, where applicable, the members of the extended family or community as provided for by local custom, legal guardians or other persons legally responsible for the child, to provide, in a manner consistent with the evolving capacities of the child, appropriate direction and guidance in the exercise by the child of the rights recognized in the present Convention."

Article 12 reads: "1. States Parties shall assure to the child who is capable of forming his or her own views the right to express those views freely in all matters affecting the child, the views of the child being given due weight in accordance with the age and maturity of the child."

Article 13 states: "1. The child shall have the right to freedom of expression; this right shall include freedom to seek, receive and impart information and ideas of all kinds, regardless of frontiers, either orally, in writing or in print, in the form of art, or through any other media of the child's choice. 2. The exercise of this right may be subject to certain restrictions, but these shall only be such as are provided by law and are necessary: (a) For respect of the rights or reputations of others; or (b) For the protection of national security or of public order (ordre public), or of public health or morals."

The issue of age, maturity, and evolving capacity is germane to the debate on adolescent harm reduction. Alcohol, cannabis, and tobacco are not treated as equal under the law. In particular, alcohol is a licit substance that is illegal for youths only by virtue of a law specifying a legal age of use access. The age for legal access to alcohol is 18 years in three Canadian provinces, 19 years in seven other provinces, 21 years in the United States, and 15 to 18 years in European countries. In 1994, Canada's Alcohol and Other Drugs Survey revealed that 74% of Canadians 15 years of age or older reported having consumed alcohol (MacNeil and Webster 1997). Notably 65% of youths 15 to 17 years of age and 80% of youths 18 to 19 years of age reported having consumed alcohol. A high percentage of adolescents attending school in Canada, the United States, and Europe have reported having consumed alcohol in the course of a year (Table 8.1). Clearly, in many jurisdictions, a majority of youths have tacitly declared themselves to be of a maturity and capacity to make decisions about alcohol consumption a few years before they have reached the legal age for consuming or buying alcohol.

It is difficult to conceive of Canadian society being rigidly intolerant of the introduction of alcohol to youths during the adolescent transition. The real issue with alcohol consumption during adolescence is that such consumption is often characterized by a high degree of risk-taking behaviour and harmful consequences, much higher than later in life. Canada's Alcohol and Other Drugs Survey inquired about alcohol-related problems in the following areas: spouse or partner, physical health, outlook on life, friendship, finances, home life, work, studies or employment, and children (MacNeil and Webster 1997). The survey revealed that 26% of current drinkers 15 to 19 years of age experienced one or more of these alcohol-related harms in the course of a year. In contrast, 10% or fewer of current drinkers 25 years of age or older experienced similar degrees of alcohol-related harm. Thus, at least in the case of alcohol, the question becomes one of how to minimize the risk of harmful consequences of alcohol use, recognizing that the majority of adolescents do use alcohol and may ignore options limited to abstinence.

Few Canadians would disagree with the message "Don't drink and drive," even, and especially, when this message is targeted to youths. The message is not an entreaty to abstain from alcohol; rather, it recognizes alcohol consumption as a personal choice but points to the risk of a specific set of harms both to the alcohol consumer and the community. Specifically, in 1995 in Canada, of the estimated 6,507 deaths attributed to alcohol consumption, the greatest percentage (18%) stemmed from impaired-driving accidents, many of which involved youths (Single et al. 2000). "Don't drink and drive" is an example of a harm reduction strategy that, despite targeting adolescents, has long since become accepted by the Canadian public.

Harm reduction pertaining to adolescent use of illicit substances remains problematic since it is unclear how a child's maturity and evolving capacity are to be judged in the case of behaviours not sanctioned for any age group in our society. The United Nations Convention is explicit in several articles that the child's rights may be limited by the demands for public order, public health, or morals. Based on the Convention, *any* harm reduction strategy addressing illicit substance use by adolescents, or use of a legal substance prior to the legal age, can be viewed as being in flagrant conflict with legal sanctions against substances, whether or not a child has achieved sufficient maturity and decision-making capacity. By contrast,

Canada's Drug Strategy does not appear to have such constraints with regard to the possible approaches to addressing adolescent substance use.

Regarding tobacco, it is difficult to see how harm reduction might apply specifically to cigarette smoking in the case of adolescents. In the four Atlantic provinces at the end of the 1990s, the prevalence of cigarette smoking among adolescents in school ranged from 27% in Prince Edward Island to 38% in Newfoundland and Labrador (Barcelo, Jones, and Grobe 1998; MacDonald and Holmes 1998; Poulin and Baker 1998; Van Til, MacMillan, and Poulin 1998). In 1995, an estimated 34,728 deaths in Canada were tobacco-related, and tobacco-attributable mortality and morbidity accounted for 16.5% of total mortality, 15.7% of total potential years of life lost, and 6.5% of all admissions to hospital (Single et al. 2000). Thus, the largest share of the economic cost of substance abuse in Canada in 1992 was associated with tobacco use rather than with alcohol or illicit drug use. The high relative risk of morbidity and mortality associated with cigarette smoking, coupled with the relatively high prevalence of cigarette smoking demonstrated by the Health Behaviour in School-aged Children survey (hbsc.org), suggests that the burden of suffering due to smoking is high in other countries as well.

The current policy imperative in Canada is for comprehensive tobacco control strategies that include taxation, legislation on smoke-free workplaces and public places, policies for smoke-free schools, prevention education, cessation programs, and, in some provinces, legal action instigated by the provincial government aimed at recovering smoking-related health care costs from the tobacco industry. Harm reduction based on nicotine replacement or maintenance therapy has been proposed and was discussed in depth at a 1997 international workshop entitled "Alternative Nicotine Delivery Systems: Harm Reduction and Public Health" (Ferrence et al. 2000). There is currently, however, no evidence about the effectiveness of such a harm reduction strategy that targets adolescents (Poulin 2000).

Clearly, harm reduction strategies targeting adolescents must be appropriate for their age, maturity, and evolving capacity, and they must address substances and their potential harms with a degree of specificity. The onus is therefore on public institutions and other custodians of adolescents to accurately judge their maturity and capacity, as individuals and as a group, relative to substance, harm, and strategy.

Out-of-the-Mainstream Youth

Not all adolescents live at home, have a home, or are under the guardianship of an adult. While not necessarily legally emancipated, many street youths would consider themselves to have the maturity and capacity to make decisions about their lives, including substance use and ways to minimize risks. Estimates of the size of the street-youth population in Canada vary widely, and indeed the numbers vary widely across urban areas (Caputo, Weiler, and Anderson 1997). A high percentage of street youths use alcohol, tobacco, and other drugs and are at high risk of serious harms, including viral hepatitis, HIV/AIDS, and death (Health and Welfare Canada 1993; Roy et al. 2001). Although not mentioned explicitly, the Convention on the Rights of the Child addresses the rights of all children and makes clear through numerous articles that States Parties must safeguard the rights of out-of-the-mainstream youth.

In general, Canadian public health and addictions services have come to consider harm reduction as an appropriate, desirable, and sometimes life-saving goal and strategy for out-of-the-mainstream adolescents. One example of a well-designed project to support such youths is the Street-Involved Youth Harm Reduction Project that took place in Toronto in 1996 (Breland, Tupker, and West 1998). The project was based on participatory research, with street-involved youths empowered to make major decisions about the direction of the project. The process evaluation revealed a sense of commitment and growth among the youths and a mutual respect between the youths and professionals working with them.

Notwithstanding the inflexibility of the Convention on the Rights of the Child relative to youth substance use, assistance and outreach to street youth with an aim to harm reduction is already an accepted part of "best practice" in Canada.

Drug Education as a Shared Responsibility of the Health and Education Systems

The Convention on the Rights of the Child identifies school as an institution that provides education, guidance, and discipline to foster personal development and good citizenship. The Convention also recognizes health care, including preventative care, as a child's right. Taken together, Articles 24, 28, and 29 of the Convention view the education and health systems as sharing responsibility for addressing drug education and prevention.

Article 24 reads: "1. States Parties recognize the right of the child to the enjoyment of the highest attainable standard of health and to facilities for the treatment of illness and rehabilitation of health ... 2. States Parties shall pursue full implementation of this right and, in particular, shall take appropriate measures: ... (f) To develop preventive health care, guidance for parents and family planning education and services."

Article 28 reads: "1. States Parties recognize the right of the child to education, and with a view to achieving this right progressively and on the basis of equal opportunity, they shall, in particular: ... (e) Take measures to encourage regular attendance at school and the reduction of drop-out rates ... 2. States Parties shall take all appropriate measures to ensure that school discipline is administered in a manner consistent with the child's human dignity and in conformity with the present Convention."

Article 29 reads: "1. States Parties agree that the education of the child shall be directed to: ... (d) The preparation of the child for responsible life in a free society, in the spirit of understanding, peace, tolerance, equality of sexes, and friendship among all peoples, ethnic, national and religious groups and persons of indigenous origin."

School dropout and discipline (Article 28) are germane to the topic of harm reduction for two reasons. First, youths out of school, either through absenteeism or school dropout, are more likely to engage in substance use behaviours (Caputo, Weiler, and Anderson 1997; Johnston and O'Malley 1985). Second, the application of disciplinary sanctions such as detention, suspension, and expulsion is thought to create further alienation and disconnection of students already feeling excluded from the school community, ultimately increasing the risk of dropout and substance use (D'Emidio-Caston and Brown 1998).

In Article 29, the mention of education that prepares the child for responsible life in a free society draws attention to two facets of harm reduction. First is the notion of personal responsibility. In the case of alcohol and tobacco, Canadians are free to choose whether to use or not use these substances. The notion of "responsible use" predates Canada's Drug Strategy (Health and Welfare Canada 1992; Health Canada 1998), and indeed some provincial addiction agencies actively advocated for responsible use, particularly regarding alcohol.

Adolescence can be viewed as a life stage during which responsible use (at least of alcohol) can be reasonably promoted. The second facet of harm reduction invoked by Article 29 pertains to the ideas of free society and societal values. In identifying harm reduction as its basic tenet, Canada's Drug Strategy tacitly accepts respect for the dignity and rights of the drug user. While harm reduction may be a philosophy with which some Canadians disagree, the National Drug Strategy (the predecessor to Canada's Drug Strategy) was adopted through an Act of Parliament in 1987 and, as such, represents values acceptable to a democratic society. Thus, this article of the Convention can be viewed as supporting harm reduction as outlined in Canada's Drug Strategy.

School-based Drug Education

We finally arrive at a major debate in the health and education fields. In which direction should school-based drug education evolve? Should the traditional focus, which is the prevention of drug use itself, be subsumed within a broader harm reduction approach?

Provincial departments of health have, over the past twenty years, implemented numerous community-based programs with a harm reduction approach. Harm reduction has generally become accepted in the addictions and health fields. In contrast, drug education in schools is largely based on the stance that substance use in any of its forms is unacceptable. As a result, school policy regarding substance use is largely punitive. Thus, there is an apparent mismatch between (a) the philosophic underpinnings of addictions programming and policy as articulated by the health system and (b) drug education as implemented by the school system.

Critical reviews of drug prevention programs have concluded that school-based primary prevention programs are largely ineffective. Although such programs increase students' knowledge, their effectiveness for preventing alcohol and other drug use per se has repeatedly been shown to be equivocal or short-lived (Bangert-Downs 1988; Brown and Horowitz 1993; Health and Welfare Canada 1992; O'Connor and Saunders 1992; Resnicow and Botvin 1993; Rundall and Bruvold 1988; Tobler 1986; White and Pitts 1998). A widespread upward trend in the prevalence of adolescent substance use was observed internationally in the 1990s (Adlaf et al. 2000; Bauman and Phongsavan 1999; Johnston, O'Malley, and Bachman 1999;

Miller and Plant 1996; Poulin et al. 1999). This upward trend has led to further doubts about the effectiveness of primary drug prevention education. One theory about the upswing is that anti-"substance use" initiatives in the 1980s were widespread and effective and that the population-level attitudinal tolerance to drugs observed in the 1990s was due to waning drug prevention efforts (Bachman, Johnston, and O'Malley 1998). An opposing theory is that drug prevention programming and policy – as it has been conceptualized and implemented – might be wrong-headed and therefore ineffective (Gorman 1998).

Increasingly, there have been calls for integrating harm reduction into school-based drug education and prevention programs (Brown and Horowitz 1993; Duncan et al. 1994; Erickson 1997; Kay 1994; Marlatt, Somers, and Tapert 1993; Poulin and Elliott 1997). Harm reduction, however, goes against established drug education practice in schools, which, at least in the United States, is rooted in a history spanning one hundred years, with strong overtones of economic, moral, and social control (Beck 1998). Furthermore, little evidence currently exists about the effectiveness of school-based harm reduction. As we demonstrate in the next section, such evidence is essential if a harm reduction approach is to be seriously considered as a valid alternative to drug prevention education.

School-Based Harm Reduction Drug Education

Erickson (1997) defines harm reduction drug education as "education about drugs rather than against drugs. The goal is to provide accurate and credible information that will promote responsible behaviour. This approach acknowledges the appeal of drug use from the young person's perspective as well as its potential medical, social and legal consequences. It is rooted in an appreciation of adolescent psycho-social development, in which curiosity, a willingness to experiment and the definition of personal boundaries come into play" (1397–1398).

An extensive review of the literature reveals few published harm reduction drug education approaches that incorporate enough of the attributes of harm reduction, document enough of the processes, and perform a formal evaluation to allow for application elsewhere. The following are projects targeting youths in school that most clearly adhere to a harm reduction philosophy.

In the United Kingdom, Cohen and his colleagues broadly disseminated a school curriculum that sought to train teachers in harm reduction drug education (Clements, Cohen, and Kay 1996; Cohen 1993; 1996; 1997; Kay 1994). The packages aimed to provide health and education professionals, parents, and students with factual information about drugs and drug use and step-by-step plain language guidelines for program and policy development, interactive activities, and parent-child discussion and problem solving. Despite the dissemination of thousands of copies in schools, colleges, youth clubs, and other settings in the United Kingdom, other than teacher satisfaction reports, the effectiveness of the approach does not appear to have been evaluated (Healthwise 1997). There is no evidence that harm reduction ultimately was achieved among adolescents.

In the United States, a school-based harm reduction demonstration project was accomplished by Somers (1995) as part of his doctoral dissertation. The research plan made explicit the psychological theories underpinning the intervention, the harm reduction goals, the methods for evaluating perceived effectiveness as well as objective impact, the intervention, and the study participants. The goals were to reduce both problems related to alcohol use and overall levels of alcohol use, to promote moderate drinking and abstinence as risk reduction options, and to evaluate students' receptiveness to the harm reduction approach. The project comprised a needs assessment and a brief cognitive-behavioural alcohol prevention intervention. The project involved only fifty students enrolled in one private school (approximately 33% of the students). The evaluation revealed: (a) a significant reduction in harmful consequences using explicit criteria and (b) no change in the baseline prevalence of alcohol abstinence. A real difficulty with this approach, however, is that, because of administrators' concerns with implementing a prevention program that was not abstinence-oriented, it would not be feasible in the public school system,.

In Canada, the Rural and Northern Youth Intervention Strategy (RNYIS) initially involved eighteen schools in twelve school districts in Manitoba (Proactive Information Services Incorporated 1994; 1995). Although the term "harm reduction" was not used in the report, the project addressed the early problem/early detection part of the risk continuum. The program used a student assistance model in which students at high risk were referred to a special Addictions Foundation of Manitoba (AFM) counsellor. Schools were required to develop comprehensive alcohol and drug policies that supported rather than punished students. The evaluation revealed that:

(a) an early intervention process had been established, but with variable implementation levels and staff ownership;
(b) collaborative interaction with community professionals had increased, but not to its full potential; and
(c) an AFM counsellor played a role in dealing with chemical dependency that could not realistically have been played by teachers.

Overall, this evaluation suggested the approach used in the project could potentially result in some harm reduction, pending improved project implementation.

Most recently, in Australia, a classroom-based harm reduction project was implemented and is being tested in fourteen urban, government secondary schools (McBride et al. 2000). The goal of the School Health and Alcohol Harm Reduction Project (SHAHRP) is to reduce alcohol-related harm by enhancing students' abilities to identify and deal with high-risk drinking situations that they are likely to encounter. This project is a well-designed, quasi-experimental study, with pre- and post-measurement of explicit harms in the intervention and control groups. The intervention is a curriculum-based program. The early results demonstrate knowledge and attitudinal change as well as lower increases in alcohol consumption among students in the intervention group in the first year of the project.

Equally interesting is the larger context of the study. Australia's National Drug Strategy has been based on harm reduction principles since 1993. The National Initiatives in Drug Education project, launched by the Australian Commonwealth Government in collaboration with the states and territories, aims to enhance school drug education in the entire country (Midford and McBride 1999). The states and territories have all adopted the national approach to harm minimization as a feature of drug education.

Clearly, there is at present little solid evidence for the superiority of harm reduction as an alternative to primary prevention for school-based drug education. From the perspective of the Convention on the Rights of the Child, important aspects of an evaluation of the effectiveness of school-based harm reduction would focus on subsequent school dropout as well as on school policy and/or discipline pertaining to substance use as outcomes of interest. In that regard, the approaches from the United Kingdom, Australia, and Manitoba appear to be promising in that school policy was incorporated as a feature of harm reduction. The Australian study is especially compelling from the perspective of child rights in that it is being conducted within the context of a coherent, comprehensive national strategy that is supportive of harm reduction.

FINAL STATEMENT

In the past, my colleagues Erickson, Elliott, and I have suggested harm reduction as a philosophy and strategy to address substance use among Canadian adolescents (Poulin and Elliott 1997; Erickson 1997). The pragmatism inherent in harm reduction necessarily demanded a simultaneous call for evidence regarding effectiveness prior to a wide adoption of harm reduction as a goal or strategy. On reflection today, that call for harm reduction was based as much on an ideological stance as on epidemiological evidence. The same can be said about the strong opinions expressed in favour of abstinence, and against harm reduction, as a goal for drug education (Mangham 2001). Of note, abstinence is a theoretical, although not necessarily a pragmatic, means of decreasing the risk of harm. A harm reduction strategy that results in a decreased prevalence of harmful consequences, but in an increased prevalence of substance use, cannot be considered entirely successful: any substance use entails risk, no matter how small.

The tension that exists between these two ideologies may in fact be desirable, especially at this early stage of our understanding of the implications of harm reduction as it applies to adolescents. Canada's Drug Strategy supports harm reduction as well as primary prevention. The United Nations Convention on the Rights of the Child recognizes both the evolving capacities of the child and the need for public order and safety. Thus, the Convention can serve to promote a necessary debate on Canada's approach to adolescent substance use, including harm reduction. Ultimately, individual and societal comfort or discomfort with harm reduction as an approach to adolescent substance use rests primarily on beliefs and values concerning the decision-making capacity of adolescents and the real harms of substance use.

REFERENCES

Adlaf, E.M., A. Paglia, F.J. Ivis, and A. Ialomiteanu. 2000. Nonmedical drug use among adolescent students: Highlights from the 1999 Ontario Student Drug Use Survey. *Canadian Medical Association Journal* 162(12):1677–80.

Ames, N.L., and E. Miller. 1994. *Changing Middle Schools: How to Make Schools Work for Young Adolescents.* San Francisco, CA: Jossey-Bass.

Bachman, J.G., L.D. Johnston, and P.M. O'Malley. 1998. Explaining recent increases in students' marijuana use: Impacts of perceived risks and disapproval, 1976 through 1996. *American Journal of Public Health* 88:887–92.

Bangert-Downs, R.L. 1988. The effects of school-based substance abuse education: A meta-analysis. *Journal of Drug Education* 18:243–64.

Barcelo, A., B. Jones, and C. Grobe. 1998. *Provincial Student Drug Use Survey: Highlights 1998.* Fredericton: New Brunswick Department of Health and Community Services, Provincial Epidemiology Service.

Bauman, A., and P. Phongsavan. 1999. Epidemiology of substance use in adolescence: Prevalence, trends and policy implications. *Drug and Alcohol Dependence* 55:187–207.

Beck, J. 1998. 100 Years of "Just Say No" versus "Just Say Know": Reevaluating drug education goals for the coming century. *Evaluation Review* 22(1):15–45.

Breland, K., E. Tupker, and P. West. 1998. *Let 'Em Go: The Street-Involved Youth Harm Reduction Project Experience.* Toronto: Centre for Addiction and Mental Health.

Brown, J.H., and J.E. Horowitz. 1993. Deviance and deviants: Why adolescent substance use prevention programs do not work. *Evaluation Review* 17(5):529–55.

Caputo, T., R. Weiler, and J. Anderson. 1997. *The Street Lifestyle Study.* Prepared for Office of Alcohol, Drugs and Dependency Issues, Health Canada. Ottawa: Minister of Public Works and Government Services Canada.

Clements, I., J. Cohen, and J. Kay. 1996. *Taking Drugs Seriously: A Manual of Harm Minimising Education on Drugs*, 3rd ed. Liverpool, UK: Healthwise.

Cohen, J. 1993. Achieving a reduction in drug related harm through education. In *Psychoactive Drugs and Harm Reduction: From Faith to Science*, ed. N. Heather, A. Wodak, E.A. Nadelmann, and P. O'Hare, 77–92. London, UK: Whurr Publishers.

– 1996. Drug education: Politics, propaganda and censorship. *International Journal on Drug Policy* 7:153–7.

– 1997. *Dealing with Drugs: An Information, Guidance and Training Manual for Drug Coordinators in Secondary and Primary Schools*, 2nd ed. Liverpool, UK: Healthwise.

D'Emidio-Caston, M., and J.H. Brown. 1998. The other side of the story: Student narratives on the California Drug, Alcohol, and Tobacco Education Programs. *Evaluation Review* 22(1):95–117.

Duncan, D.F., T. Nicholson, P. Clifford, W. Hawkins, and R. Petosa. 1994. Harm reduction: An emerging new paradigm for drug education. *Journal of Drug Education* 24(4):281–90.

Erickson, P.G. 1997. Reducing the harm of adolescent substance use. *Canadian Medical Association Journal* 156(10):1397–1399.

Ferrence, R., J. Slade, R. Room, and M. Pope, eds. 2000. *Nicotine and Public Health*. Washington: American Public Health Association.

Gorman, D.M. 1998. The irrelevance of evidence in the development of school-based drug prevention policy, 1986–1996. *Evaluation Review* 22(1):118–46.

Hall, W., and N. Solowij. 1998. Adverse effects of cannabis. *Lancet* 352(9140):1611–1616.

Health and Welfare Canada. 1992. *The Effectiveness of Prevention and Treatment Programs for Alcohol and Other Drugs Problems: A Review of Evaluation Studies*. A Canada's Drug Strategy Baseline Report. Ottawa: Minister of Supply and Services Canada.

– 1993. *A Study of Out-of-the-Mainstream Youth in Halifax, Nova Scotia: Technical Report*. Ottawa: Minister of Supply and Services Canada.

Health Canada. 1998. *Canada's Drug Strategy*. Ottawa: Health Canada, Office of Alcohol, Drugs, and Dependency Issues. http://www.hc-sc.gc.ca/hppb/alcohol-otherdrugs/pdf/englishstrategy.pdf. Retrieved 1 August 2006.

Healthwise. 1997. *Schools Support Unit Annual Report, April 1996–March 1997*. Liverpool, UK: Healthwise.

Johnston, L.D., and P.M. O'Malley. 1985. Issues of validity and population coverage in student surveys of drug use. In *Self-Report Methods of Estimating Drug Use: Meeting Current Challenges to Validity*, ed. B.A. Rouse, N.J. Kozel, and L.G. Richards. NIDA Research Monograph 57. Washington, DC: National Institute on Drug Abuse (NIDA).

Johnston, L.D., P.M. O'Malley, and J.G. Bachman. 1999. National survey results on drug use from the Monitoring the Future Study,

1975–1998. In *Volume 1: Secondary School Students*. NIH Publication No. 99–4660. Washington, DC: US Department of Health and Human Services.

Kay, J. 1994. Don't wait until it's too late. *International Journal of Drug Policy* 5(3):166–75.

MacDonald, C.A., and P.R. Holmes. 1998. *Newfoundland and Labrador Student Drug Use 1998: Technical Report*. St John's: Government of Newfoundland and Labrador, Department of Health, Addictions Services.

MacNeil, P., and I. Webster. 1997. *Canada's Alcohol and Other Drugs Survey 1994: A Discussion of the Findings*. Ottawa: Health Canada.

Mangham, C. 2001. Harm reduction and illegal drugs: The real debate. *Canadian Journal of Public Health* 92(3):204–5.

Marlatt, G.A., J.M. Somers, and S.F. Tapert. 1993. Harm reduction: Application to alcohol abuse problems. In *Behavioral Treatments for Drug Abuse and Dependence*, ed. Lisa Simon Onken, Jack D. Blaine, and John J. Boren, 147–66. NIDA Research Monograph 137. Washington, DC: National Institute on Drug Abuse (NIDA).

McBride, N., R. Midford, F. Farringdon, and M. Phillips. 2000. Early results from a school alcohol harm minimization study: The School Health and Alcohol Harm Reduction Project. *Addiction* 95(7):1021–42.

McCreary Centre Society. 1999. *Healthy Connections: Listening to BC Youth*. Burnaby, BC: McCreary Centre Society.

Midford, R., and N. McBride. 1999. Evaluation of a national school drug education program in Australia. *International Journal of Drug Policy* 10:177–93.

Miller, P.McC., and M. Plant. 1996. Drinking, smoking and illicit drug use among 15 and 16 year olds in the United Kingdom. *British Medical Journal* 313:394–399.

O'Connor, J., and B. Saunders. 1992. Drug education: An appraisal of a popular preventive. *International Journal of Addictions* 27(2):165–85.

Patton, D., D. Brown, B. Broszeit, and J. Dhaliwal. 2001. *Substance Use among Manitoba High School Students*. Winnipeg: Addictions Foundation of Manitoba. http://www.afm.mb.ca/Research/documents/HSSU.pdf. Retrieved 1 August 2007.

Poulin, C. 1997. *Canadian Community Epidemiology Network on Drug Use: Inaugural National Report*. Ottawa: Canadian Centre on Substance Abuse.

– 2000. The public health implications of adopting a harm-reduction approach to nicotine. In *Nicotine and Public Health*, ed. R. Ferrence,

J. Slade, R. Room, and M. Pope. Washington: American Public Health Association.

Poulin, C., and J. Baker. 1998. *Nova Scotia Student Drug Use 1998: Technical Report*. Halifax: Nova Scotia Department of Health and Dalhousie University.

Poulin, C., and D. Elliott. 1997. Alcohol, tobacco and cannabis use among Nova Scotia adolescents: Implications for prevention and harm reduction. *Canadian Medical Association Journal* 156(10):1387–93.

Poulin, C., J. Stein, and J. Butt. 1998. Surveillance of drug overdose deaths using medical examiner data. *Chronic Diseases in Canada* 19(4):177–82.

Poulin, C., L. Van Til, B. Wilbur, B. Clarke, C.A. MacDonald, A. Barcelo, and L. Lethbridge. 1999. Alcohol and other drug use among adolescent students in the Atlantic provinces. *Canadian Journal of Public Health* 90(1):27–9.

Proactive Information Services Incorporated. 1994. *Rural and Northern Youth Intervention Strategy (RNYIS) Project Evaluation: Second Interim Report*. Prepared for Addictions Foundation of Manitoba. Winnipeg: Proactive Information Services Incorporated.

– 1995. *Rural and Northern Youth Intervention Strategy (RNYIS) Project Evaluation: Final Report*. Prepared for Addictions Foundation of Manitoba. Winnipeg: Proactive Information Services Incorporated.

Resnicow, K., and G. Botvin. 1993. School-based substance use prevention programs: Why do effects decay? *Preventive Medicine* 22:484–90.

Riley, D., E. Sawka, P. Conley, D. Hewitt, W. Mitic, C. Poulin, R. Room, E. Single, and J. Topp. 1999. Harm reduction: Concepts and practice. A policy discussion paper. *Substance Use and Misuse* 34(1):9–24.

Roy, E., N. Haley, P. Leclerc, J.F. Boivin, L. Cedras, and J. Vincelette. 2001. Risk factors for hepatitis C virus infection among street youths. *Canadian Medical Association Journal* 165:557–660.

Rundall, T.G, and W.H. Bruvold. 1988. A meta-analysis of school-based smoking and alcohol use prevention programs. *Health Education Quarterly* 15:317–44.

Single, E., J. Rehm, L. Robson, and M.V. Truong. 2000. The relative risks and etiologic fractions of different causes of death and disease attributable to alcohol, tobacco and illicit drug use in Canada. *Canadian Medical Association Journal* 162(12):1669–75.

Somers, J. 1995. Harm reduction and the prevention of alcohol problems among secondary school students. Phd dissertation, Seattle, University of Washington.

Tobler, N.S. 1986. Meta-analysis of 143 adolescent drug prevention programs: Quantitative outcome results of program participants compared to a control or comparison group. *Journal of Drug Issues* 16:537–67.

United Nations. 1989. *Convention on the Rights of the Child.* Geneva: United Nations.

Van Til, L., H. MacMillan, and C. Poulin. 1998. *Prince Edward Island Student Drug Use 1998: Technical Report.* Charlottetown, PEI: Department of Health and Social Services.

White, D., and M. Pitts. 1998. Educating young people about drugs: A systematic review. *Addiction* 93(10):1475–87.

9

Responding to Bullying and Harassment: An Issue of Rights

DEBRA PEPLER AND WENDY CRAIG

INTRODUCTION

Over the past decade and a half, there has been increased concern about violence among youth. Not only adults, but youths themselves feel concerned for their safety and security (King, Boyce, and King 1999). The response to this concern within the justice and educational systems has been to establish increasingly severe sanctions for young offenders. At the same time, there has been a paucity of attention to the rights, protection, and support of victimized youths. In this chapter, we review research that highlights the nature of abuse, such as bullying, that adolescents experience at the hands of their peers. From this research, we draw implications for rights-based social policies that both protect victims of peer abuse and support the healthy development of all aggressive youths. Such policies should be comprehensive and their development and implementation should involve not only researchers and policy-makers but also those youths who are victimized, those who bully, their peers, parents, schools, and communities.

BACKGROUND

Definition of Bullying and Harassment

Bullying is one type of peer harassment that can take different forms at different ages. Bullying is defined as repeated aggression in which there is a power differential (Juvonen and Graham 2001; Olweus 1991; Pepler and Craig 2000). Two elements of bullying are key to understanding its complexity. First, bullying is a form of aggressive behaviour effected from a position of power: children who bully always have more power than their victims. Anyone in a position of relative power – children, youths, or adults – has the potential to bully others. This power can derive from a physical advantage such as size, age, and strength, but power can also be acquired through a social advantage such as a dominant social role (e.g., teacher compared to student), higher social status in a peer group (e.g., popular versus rejected student), or through strength in numbers (e.g., a group of adolescents picking on a solitary student). Power can be achieved through knowing another's source of vulnerability (e.g., obesity, stuttering, learning problem, family background) and using that knowledge to cause distress. The second key element is that bullying is repeated over time. With each repeated bullying incident, the power relations between the bully and victim become consolidated: the bully increases in power and the victim loses power. In a relationship that has developed in this way, the adolescent who is being bullied becomes powerless to solve the problem by him- or herself.

Bullying can take many forms. It can be physical (e.g., hits, pushes, trips, spitting), verbal (e.g., threats, taunts, insults, putdowns), and social (e.g., social exclusion, malicious gossip) or cyber (e.g., malicious text messages, destructive websites, spreading rumours through e-mail). Bullying may be direct: for example, the adolescent who is being victimized is confronted by the aggressive youth(s). It can also be indirect: for example, of youths may plot to create a distressing event without confronting the victimized youth and revealing their identity (e.g., starting a rumour, creating an embarrassing situation).

Developmental Perspective:
Changes in Bullying and Harassment with Age

The nature of bullying changes as youths mature. In early adolescence and beyond, new forms of aggression, carried out from a position of power, emerge. With their developing cognitive and social skills, adolescents become increasingly aware of others' vulnerabilities and of their power relative to others. Therefore, with age, bullying diversifies into more sophisticated forms of verbal and social aggression as well as into sexually and racially based aggression.

Diversification in the form of bullying is consistent with the developmental theory of aggressive strategies postulated by Bjorkqvist and his colleagues (1992). Their data on aggressive strategies reveal that, as verbal skills and social intelligence develop, there is a move away from using physically aggressive strategies and an increased tendency to use verbal and indirect (socially manipulative) strategies (Bjorkqvist, Osterman, and Kaukiainen 1992). In our research on bullying, we recognize that the form of bullying that youths use will reflect the challenges of their developmental stage.

Bullying and harassment transform according to the changing sensitivities and vulnerabilities of the individuals being victimized. In early adolescence, pubertal changes occur and youths become increasingly sensitive about their emerging sexuality and sexual orientation. During this period, the prevalence of sexual harassment increases; those adolescents prone to bullying are at greater risk for sexually harassing their peers compared to youths who do not exhibit patterns of power and aggression (McMaster et al., 2002). In adolescence, multiple aspects of identity are in the process of consolidation; therefore, attacks based on sexual orientation or racial background strike at the core of the developing self. Throughout the lifespan, bullying and harassment encompass malicious comments and behaviours related to sexuality, race, disability, disadvantage, and difference. The key factor required in identifying bullying and harassment is whether this behaviour is "unwelcomed." A behaviour that is not troublesome to one youth may be extremely hurtful to another because of that youth's individual vulnerabilities and identity.

With an increasing ability to understand what others are thinking (theory of mind), adolescents who bully are able to determine what comments or behaviours will cause significant distress to their victims (Sutton, Smith, and Swettenham 1999). This knowledge gives adolescents a basis of power relative to others. Although they often do not acknowledge bullying, a substantial proportion of high school students report that they sexually harass others (McMaster et al. 1998). A smaller proportion report being engaged in gang behaviour (both formal and informal) and aggression with dating partners (Pepler et al. 2001). These problem behaviours share the combination of power and aggression that defines bullying and are a problem throughout the lifespan, manifesting themselves in malicious comments and behaviours related to sexuality, race, disability, disadvantage, and difference. Youths do not just grow out of bullying; on the contrary, we are concerned that adolescents who learn how to acquire power through aggression on the playground may transfer these lessons to sexual harassment, date violence, gang attacks, marital abuse, child abuse, and elder abuse, all of which have significant financial and social costs (Farrington 1993).

The Prevalence of Bullying

Bullying is a problem that transcends national boundaries and appears to unfold in many cultures, although the concept of bullying is not universal. A recent multinational study examined the definition of bullying and found that the words chosen to represent "bullying" on questionnaires may influence the number of youths who respond that they have perpetrated or been victimized by bullying (Smith et al. 2002). Taking this cross-national variability into consideration, data from the World Health Organization (WHO) survey of Health Behaviour in School-aged Children (HBSC) provide a perspective on the safety of Canadian students' relationships.

In the last report from the HBSC study, with thirty-five countries participating including Canada, the survey assessed a wide range of behaviours, including bullying, among 11-, 13- and 15-year-old students. In the ranking with other countries on the 2001/2002 survey, Canada's position on the prevalence of bullying and victimization was dismal. For example, among 13-year-old children, 17.8% of boys and 11.6% of girls bullied others frequently (twice or more), while 17.8% of boys and 15.1% of girls were victimized frequently (Craig and Harel 2005). Canada ranked twenty-sixth and twenty-seventh out of the thirty-five countries on bullying and victimization, respectively. Across all ages and frequency categories of bullying or victimization, Canada consistently ranks at or below the middle of the international group. Our position on the international stage has slipped relative to other countries. On the 1993/1994 survey, Canada's ranking on the prevalence of bullying and victimization was much higher compared to the other twenty-five participating nations than was the case in the 2001/2002 survey (King et al. 1996). Over this eight-year period, the prevalence rates of bullying and victimization among Canadian students have remained relatively stable. The drop in Canada's ranking, in spite of the relatively stable rates, suggests that other countries have been addressing bullying problems more effectively than Canada. Many of the countries that

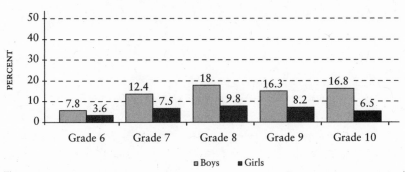

Figure 9.1
Prevalence of bullying

rank higher than Canada have had national campaigns to address bullying problems. Although there are many Canadian activities at local, provincial, and national levels to prevent and reduce the risks of bullying and victimization, they tend to use diverse assessment and intervention tools; they are not rigorously evaluated, and they operate in isolation without an evidence-based national platform for coordination and implementation.

Although a substantial number of youths are occasionally involved in bullying and victimization, a small group of youths frequently bully others or are bullied by peers (Craig and Pepler 1997; Olweus 1993; Leff et al. 1999). These are the youths who are likely in need of focused support to enable them to move on from these abusive interactions with peers, either as the perpetrator or the victim (Pepler and Craig 2000). Using the WHO Canadian HBSC data for children in grades 6 to 10, we categorized adolescents as bullies or victims if they indicated that they had bullied another student or been bullied by another student in school "sometimes," "about once a week," or "several times a week" during the term. This research was inclusive in its definition of bullying, including physical, verbal, direct, and indirect forms of aggressive behaviour. The following figures reflect the percentage of adolescents who indicated they had bullied, had been bullied, or had been both a bully and a victim during the term.

We start by examining the prevalence of bullying with data from boys and girls in grades 6 to 10. As can be seen from Figure 9.1, boys are more likely than girls to report perpetrating bullying across all grades. With age there is an increase in bullying, with a peak for boys and girls in grade 8. In grade 10, one in six boys and one in

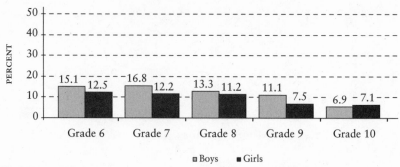

Figure 9.2
Prevalence of victimization

twenty-five girls is willing to acknowledge that they bully others
sometimes or more often at school. Youths who bully others are
more likely to use drugs and alcohol, smoke, and have low self-
esteem compared to youths who do not bully (Craig, Goldbaum, et
al. 2001). They also have poorer quality of relationships with their
families, more anti-social peers, and more negative attitudes towards
school compared to youths who do not engage in bullying (Boivin,
Hymel, and Hodges 2001; Craig, Goldbaum, et al. 2001; Perry,
Hodges, and Egan 2001).

The prevalence for victimization of boys and girls in grades 6 to
10 is illustrated in Figure 9.2. The gender differences in victimization
are not as dramatic as those for bullying. Boys report significantly
more victimization than girls in grades 7 and 9, but there are no
significant gender differences in grades 6, 8, and 10. The peak in
reports of victimization appears in grade 7, with a gradual decrease
in bullying through the early and mid-adolescent years. Nevertheless,
in grade 10, over one in twenty students is still experiencing bullying
by peers on a regular basis at school. Youths who are victimized
tend to report low self-esteem and low-quality friendships and family
relationships compared to youths who are not victimized by others
(Craig, Goldbaum, et al. 2001).

Numerous studies have indicated that a small proportion of youths
are involved both as perpetrators and victims of bullying (Craig and
Pepler 1997; Schwartz, Proctor, and Chien 2001). These youths are
frequently involved in conflict with their peers. As Figure 9.3 illustrates, a small proportion of boys and girls report they both bully
others and are victimized. As with victimization, the gender differences in bully/victim reports are inconsistent across grades. Significantly

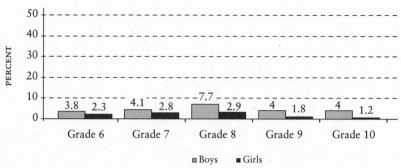

Figure 9.3
Prevalence of bullying and victimization

more boys than girls report both bullying and victimization in grades 8, 9, and 10; however, there are not significant differences among the younger adolescents in grades 6 and 7. The peak for the prevalence of bully-victim classifications is in grade 8 for both boys and girls. Even though these percentages of youths are small, these are the students who are at highest risk for a range of emotional and behavioural problems (Pepler, Craig, and Connolly 1997).

WHY WORRY ABOUT BULLYING AND HARASSMENT?

These prevalence data indicate that a substantial proportion of youths are involved in bullying as the aggressor and/or as the victim. There is reason to be concerned about adolescents involved in bullying and harassment interaction. They are at risk for long-term problems with anti-social behaviour and substance use (Farrington 1993; Huesmann et al. 1984; Olweus 1991). Victimized youths are also at risk for anxiety, depression, and somatic complaints (Olweus 1992; Rigby 2001). To prevent these negative long-term outcomes, we need to support adolescents' healthy development and protect their welfare at the same time as engaging with them in finding a solution to the problem. This requirement is identified in the United Nations Convention on the Rights of the Child (UNCRC) (United Nations 1989). In Article 29, the Convention specifies that education shall be directed to "[t]he preparation of the child for responsible life in a free society, in the spirit of understanding, peace, tolerance, equality of sexes, and friendship among all peoples, ethnic, national and religious groups and persons of indigenous origin." Therefore, it is the role of society to involve and educate youths to ensure they develop positive attitudes and behaviours and avoid using their power to bully or harass others. This societal function is the responsibility of parents, teachers, and other adults in the community who are in contact with children and youth.

The UN Convention on the Rights of the Child also speaks to the rights of youths who are at the receiving end of bullying and harassment. Article 19 of the Convention asserts: "States Parties shall take all appropriate legislative, administrative, social and educational measures to protect the child from all forms of physical or mental violence, injury or abuse, neglect or negligent treatment, maltreatment or exploitation, including sexual abuse, while in the care of parent(s), legal guardian(s) or any other person who has the care of the child."

Traditionally, the definition of child abuse has been limited to abuse perpetrated by an adult. Recently, research on bullying has highlighted the need to expand this definition to include the torment that some youths experience at the hands of their peers (cf. Juvonen and Graham 2001). For every youth concerned about being sexually abused by adults, there are three children concerned about being beaten up by peers (Finkelhor, Assdigan, and Dziuba-Leatherman 1995). Recent research on the negative effects of peer harassment (cf. Juvonen and Graham 2001) underlines the importance of protecting youths from "all forms of physical or mental violence, injury or abuse" perpetrated by peers. This societal responsibility falls to parents, teachers, and other adults and must involve youths themselves.

UNDERSTANDING ADOLESCENT DEVELOPMENT AND DEVELOPING EFFECTIVE INTERVENTIONS

Understanding the mechanisms that promote adolescent development is critical to the development of effective interventions (American Psychological Association 2001). From the determinants of health perspective on addressing bullying and victimization problems, it is essential to recognize that youth development is shaped by multiple interacting factors, including their individual predispositions, family, school environments, peer groups, and broader communities (Ford and Lerner 1992). Numerous factors within these domains have been identified as risk factors for bullying and/or victimization. Not all youths with these characteristics will become bullies or victims:

their developmental course is shaped by their interactions within social contexts such as the family, peer group, and school. With an understanding of these risk factors within multiple domains, we can assess, intervene, and follow-up to support youths who are vulnerable to becoming aggressive or victimized. No youth is destined to become a bully or a victim, but a combination of risk factors within the youth and within his or her environment create a vulnerability to becoming a bully or a victim. Within each developmental stage (e.g., infancy, childhood, adolescence, adulthood), there are both specific and non-specific risk factors. Adolescence is a period of dramatic biological and social changes, with puberty and maturation accompanied by changes in the family and peer relationships. We turn now to a discussion of these risk factors in adolescence within our systemic perspective.

Individual Characteristics of the Adolescent

In the transition to adolescence, the biological changes of puberty exert a major influence on development. Of particular importance are variations in the timing and onset of pubertal changes. These variations are associated with both bullying and victimization (Craig, Pepler, et al. 2001). For bullies, early onset of puberty may serve to maintain their power over peers. Conversely, both early and late onset of puberty may be associated with victimization if it distinguishes a student from their peer group in an obvious manner. The biological changes of adolescence also influence the content of bullying. In this time, emerging sexuality is salient as youths move into mixed-sex peer groups and romantic relationships. Since sexuality is a highly sensitive topic to young adolescents, victimization around sexual issues has high potential for causing distress, especially for early-maturing or late-maturing youths. In our own data, we found that early-developing boys and girls were more likely to experience significantly more same- and opposite-sex sexual harassment than their on-time peers (Craig, Pepler, et al. 2001).

A second individual risk factor for victimization is prior involvement in bullying or victimization. Youths' experiences with bullying and victimization will shape their responses in the future. Aggressive behaviour is a relatively stable behaviour over time (Huesmann et al. 1984; Olweus 1993). Retrospective research confirms that, for boys, victimization is relatively stable from childhood to adulthood

(Olweus 1994). Our observational research indicates that victimized youths often respond to interpersonal attacks with maladaptive coping styles (Mahady-Wilton, Craig, and Pepler 2000). We suggest that, over time, both those children who bully and those who are victimized may develop an increasingly negative reputation within the peer group, and peers may become increasingly reluctant to associate with them for fear of being victimized themselves (Craig and Pepler 1995).

Family Factors

Families provide the primary socialization experiences for youths who learn how to relate to others and how to solve conflicts through their experiences at home. Youths who grow up in an aggressive home, with parents who are not effective in discouraging aggression and promoting pro-social behaviors, are at risk for transferring the lessons in aggression to their peer and school interactions (Patterson, DeBaryshe, and Ramsey 1989). Sibling interactions have the potential to contribute to the risk of bullying or victimization. Patterson (1986) articulated how aggressive youths regularly engage in fighting with their siblings and how siblings contribute directly to the coercive processes that train youths in aggressive strategies. Less is known about the role of family characteristics, including family structure, income, and education, of youths who are victimized. Youths may be at risk for victimization if their parents are over-protective and prevent them from encountering developmental challenges normal for their stage (Perry, Hodges, and Egan 2001). Experiences of victimization by siblings may transfer to interactions with peers, but at this point these risks are speculative.

Peer Factors

After the family, the peer group is a central socializing domain for youths. In adolescence, youths spend less time with their families and more time with peers. The time that they spend with peers tends to be unsupervised by adults, and there is an increase in peer influence during this phase. Thus, peers provide an important context for the development of bullying. In our observational research, we found that peers were present in 85% of bullying episodes on the school playground (Craig and Pepler 1997). Peers who observe bullying engage in many behaviours that reinforce bullies for their aggressive and dominant behaviours (O'Connell, Pepler, and Craig 1999). These dynamics within the peer group contribute to the risk for bullying, particularly if youths associate with other aggressive youths and have few interactions with their pro-social peers (Dishion, McCord, and Poulin 1999). Youths who are generally disliked within their peer group and have few or no friends are at risk for being victimized (Hodges et al. 1999). Without friends, these youths are unlikely to be supported by peers who might intervene to stop bullying (Hawkins, Pepler, and Craig 2001).

As adolescents shift to spending more time with peers and less time with their families, there may be more opportunities for bullying to occur in the community. When groups of anti-social youths aggregate in unsupervised settings, the likelihood of adult intervention to stop bullying is low and the potential for harm is high.

Adolescent social interactions are shaped by the biological changes described above. Adolescents' emerging sexuality underlies the social change from same-sex peer groups to mixed-sex peer groups (Connolly et al. 1999). These biological and social changes, in turn, shift the context, so that bullying and victimization move from being enacted by a member of the same-sex peer group to being enacted by a cross-sex peer. The use of power and aggression may also unfold in the romantic relationships of youths who tend to bully their peers (Connolly et al. 2000).

School Factors

Interactions within the school environment, as one example of community-level influences, can serve either to exacerbate or to correct bullying problems. Youths are likely to be more aggressive and involved in bullying if school staff ignore anti-social behaviour, provide inconsistent sanctions for bullying, and do not engage positively with troubled children. Our observations of bullying on the playground indicate that adults seldom intervene in bullying episodes (Craig and Pepler 1997). When there is little monitoring and few consequences for bullying, youths will quickly learn that they can bully others without recourse. Similarly, youths will be at risk for victimization in schools where there is a general lack of recognition of bullying problems and a lack of communication and openness about bullying and victimization (Sharpe and Smith 1994).

School is a context in which adults are responsible for promoting healthy development and ensuring that students are safe, both physically and psychologically. In this context, it is essential that students learn positive conflict resolution skills and have opportunities for positive leadership to ensure a healthy peer culture. The high school context for adolescents provides more autonomy and less monitoring than does the elementary school context. In high school, teachers are responsible for a large number of students for a short time period each day within the confines of the classroom. Because of the number of students, frequent class changes, and low monitoring, there may be more opportunities for bullying in high school than in elementary school. As a consequence, adolescents' bullying behaviours and experiences of victimization may go unnoticed.

EFFECTIVE INTERVENTIONS: SYSTEMIC PERSPECTIVE

Given that the risk for bullying and victimization can be attributed to multiple factors within the young person, family, peer group, and school, we believe that these problems must be addressed within a systemic perspective and that action must be taken on multiple levels. Interventions need to be carried out not only with regard to the adolescents who bully and are victimized but also within the school, within the peer group, and with parents. The following principles of this systemic approach are important to remember when addressing bullying and victimization.

- The earlier we support troubled youths, the less intensive and expensive the interventions for bullying and victimization need to be.
- Bullying and victimization do not occur in isolation. Therefore, interventions with the youths who bully and/or who are victimized are necessary but not sufficient.
- We need to extend our focus beyond those who bully and are victimized to include: peers, school, parents, community, and society.
- To address the problem effectively, change is required at all of these levels of the system.
- Implementing a bullying prevention program is a complex and prolonged process because of the systemic nature of the problem and its solutions.

• Leadership from the adults in youths' lives is essential to addressing bullying problems. As youths mature, this leadership can be increasingly shared with peers.

The Central Role of Adults in Addressing Bullying

The UN Convention on the Rights of the Child indicates that, while children, including adolescents, are in the care of parents, guardians, or other responsible adults, they are to be protected from all forms of abuse. Adults are also responsible for children's education to promote healthy development and citizenship. Therefore, changes in youths' lives and social contexts begin with adults. This tenet applies particularly to interventions addressing bullying and victimization. At home, parents are responsible for their adolescent's safety. When these youths go to school, it is the adults in the school who are responsible for the safety of the students. Thus, in addressing problems of bullying and victimization, both parents and educators need to take responsibility for the intervention and ensure the safety of all youth. At the same time, adults need to work actively with youths to ensure their participation in addressing bullying.

There are many challenges inherent in preventing and intervening in bullying problems. First, the subtleness and power differential in bullying make it a particularly difficult form of aggressive behaviour to detect and address. Sometimes adults are not able to determine whether a behaviour is "unwelcomed" in adolescents' interactions. From our observational studies, we found that one of the most prevalent emotions portrayed by both groups was joy or positive affect (Mahady-Wilton et al. 2000). When asked, youths who are accused of bullying will sometimes respond that "it was just in fun." The victimized youth, working from a powerless position, will often agree. Youths who are repeatedly bullied or harassed are acutely aware of the possible retaliations for identifying a bullying peer as troublesome.

Adults often fail to recognize the ways in which youths have acquired power over others. Youths who have power and choose to use it aggressively usually recognize that adults do not approve of aggressive behaviour and develop a diverse repertoire of behaviours to avoid detection. A bully-victim relationship develops over time: each time a bullying youth is successful in causing distress to the victimized youth, the youth who is bullying gains in relative power and the victimized youth loses power in the relationship. When bullying has unfolded over weeks or months, the aggressive individual need only gesture subtly to communicate that the other should be fearful of what might ensue. Adults seldom recognize these subtle gestures as aggressive behaviours. It is important, therefore, that teachers, parents, and other adults in contact with adolescents observe and listen carefully when they express concerns about bullying.

To overcome this challenge of detection of bullying, adults need education and training as part of a bullying prevention initiative. Such initiatives could involve: (a) development of assessment tools to identify areas of the playground or school where bullying is likely to occur, (b) increased supervision of these identified areas, (c) development of increased sensitivity to students' distress, and (d) teaching of prevention actions for youths being bullied (such as approaching groups of other youths who may come together). Elements of these strategies have been included in interventions around the world (Smith, Pepler, and Rigby 2004).

A second challenge relates to interventions to support youths who are bullying their peers. Not only are bullying episodes hard to detect but adults' attitudes may militate against interventions. If adults assume that "bullying is just a normal part of growing up" or that "bullying isn't serious – it's just kids being kids," then they are less likely to intervene. Our observations indicate that youths who are bullying others seldom receive corrective intervention from adults. In elementary school playgrounds and in classrooms, we observed that teachers intervened in 4% and 14% of the episodes, respectively (Atlas and Pepler 1998; Craig and Pepler 1997; Craig, Pepler, and Atlas 2000). Consequently within the school context, youths who bully others are at risk for learning that aggression from a position of power can be effective and has few negative consequences.

A final challenge for adults comes in recognizing and responding to the dynamics of bullying in order to support the youths who are victimized. The power differential that is consolidated through multiple repeated bullying episodes eventually renders victimized students powerless to defend themselves. Youths who are bullied respond in the best way they can each time they are victimized (e.g., they ignore, walk away, state their annoyance, use humour, seek others with whom to play). If these responses are successful, the bullying generally stops. For some youths in some situations, none of the strategies they try is adequate to deter the aggressor, who gains power and often excitement from the repeated bullying attacks. When youths are totally defeated and frustrated by the ongoing bullying, they may finally reach out to an adult for help. If that adult dismisses the report (e.g., saying "your glasses are fine"; "you are not fat or stupid") and tells the youth to solve the problem him- or herself (e.g., saying "use your words"; "just ignore them"), then the adult has failed to provide the essential protection and support for the youth's safety.

Systemic, whole-school interventions are increasingly demonstrated to be effective in reducing bullying problems (Olweus 1991; Pepler et al. 1994; Pepler et al. 2004; Smith, Pepler, and Rigby 2004). The process of change, however, is demanding and slow, because it requires effective interventions with the youths who bully, the youths who are victimized, the peer group, teachers, parents, and the wider community. Even the most effective interventions, such as those implemented in Norway, manage to reduce the level of bullying and victimization only by about 50% (Olweus 1991; 1993). This level of effectiveness means that many youths are still at risk for regular abuse at the hands of their peers, and many aggressive youths are not being supported to move off their troubled pathways. At this point, the solutions are within our grasp, if we can find ways of linking current social policies to research.

Policy Implications: Stopping Bullying and Harassment

The solution to the problems of bullying and harassment requires a systemic response that includes not only the bullying and victimized youths but also others in the youths' lives. The UN Convention on the Rights of the Child specifies that children should be protected from abusive experiences. Within Canada, there are laws that protect all citizens from abuse. Why then does bullying continue and why are so many youths involved in this form of peer abuse? One answer may be that it is only recently that we have recognized the significant long-term consequences of peer harassment and that we have not yet fully developed educational, social, and legal responses with health-promoting, systematic interventions. This omission serves to put both youths who bully and those who are victimized at continuing risk for psychosocial problems. Paradoxically, an approach to bullying that suggests that it is "just kids being kids" and "an important lesson to toughen up" has created a dilemma: we have laws and harassment policies that appear to protect adults to a greater extent than they protect youths, at least when it comes to peer harassment.

From a prevention and early intervention perspective, the policies governing responses to harassment (sexual, racial, etc.) among adults provide an excellent framework upon which to build an effective approach to protecting adolescents who are abused by their peers. By implementing parallel policies, we can develop schools and communities as places in which all members feel safe and are treated with respect. If a policy for addressing peer harassment is to be adequate, then it must include five basic elements: (1) a clear definition of bullying and harassment, (2) clear contextual parameters, (3) a clear statement of concern and commitment to resolve problems of bullying and harassment, (4) clear procedures and processes to resolve concerns of bullying and harassment, and (5) specified formative consequences for the children or youths who have been perpetrating the bullying or harassment. These elements are discussed below.

DEFINITION OF BULLYING AND HARASSMENT

A clear definition of bullying and harassment is essential in a policy designed to protect aggressive and victimized children. The definition must encompass both direct and indirect physical, verbal, social, and cyber bullying, and it must recognize developmental changes in bullying. The definition should extend to sexual harassment, racial harassment, and derogatory behaviours and comments based on disadvantage or difference. It should highlight the critical features of a power differential that increases with repeated bullying interactions. Experiences that are "unwelcomed" because they cause distress to the victim should be identified as bullying and harassment, thereby recognizing the inherent distress of the victim.

CONTEXTUAL PARAMETERS OF THE POLICY

A policy on bullying and harassment should set the parameters for interactions among children, youth, and adults throughout the community. It is essential that the definition and restrictions relating to bullying and harassment apply to all members of the community, whether these include a school, a team, a recreation centre, a camp, or other youth organization. Adults, who, by definition, are in a position of power relative to youth in all of these contexts, must be extremely cautious of not abusing their power through bullying and harassment.

STATEMENT OF CONCERN AND COMMITMENT

The policy must alert everyone within the community to concerns about bullying and harassment and ensure a strong commitment to respond to these problems when they are uncovered. Communication is the key to identifying bullying and harassment. Youths who are victimized, as well as peers who observe bullying and harassment, must be encouraged to intervene positively and/or to report the problem to an adult. There are barriers, however, to open communication regarding these problems. Youths fear retaliation from those who bullied them; disclosing prolonged victimization is perceived as shameful; and adults often dismiss the reports as only minor problems. It is critical to direct attention to the victimized adolescents' distress and to ensure them of the commitment to protect them from further abuse. When trying to untangle a bullying situation, it is essential that adults listen carefully to what the youths are telling them about the experiences of victimization and to put themselves in their shoes. It is only through sensitive attending that adults can begin to understand the extent of the victimized youth's distress.

PROCEDURES AND PROCESSES TO RESOLVE BULLYING AND HARASSMENT PROBLEMS

Policies need to specify strategies for assessing the problem, for implementing the procedures, and for following up after an incident has taken place. A bullying and harassment policy defines the expectations, roles, and responsibilities of all members within a community for each of these tasks. Although all members of the community should be concerned and should address issues of peer harassment, a specification of individual roles and responsibilities ensures commitment and action to support those youths involved. The youths who experience victimization or who witness it must have access to an identified and sensitized adult who is prepared to receive reports of unwelcomed behaviours. This adult must be able to assess the degree of distress and potential risk for the victimized youth. The youth's risk can be determined by assessing how severe the bullying is, how long it has been occurring, how frequently it occurs, and how pervasive it is (see Pepler and Craig 2000). Depending on the severity of the problem, the identified adult will follow one of several procedures to support the victim and to report the perpetrator. In the case of minor bullying, the interventions on the part of trained adults may be as simple as listening attentively, reviewing the youth's responses, coaching the youth in assertive responding, and establishing a follow-up strategy to ensure that the bullying has stopped. When bullying is serious and the youth is at high risk for continuing distress, procedures must be implemented to ensure that the bullying stops. The strategies adopted to support the victimized youth may include many of the systems in which the youth lives: the family, the peer group, the school, and perhaps the community beyond the setting in which the bullying occurred. The procedures adopted should not further victimize the youth by removing him or her from the context in which the bullying occurs (e.g., school, sports team). An assessment of the victim's vulnerability and potential strengths will help in formulating plans for building her/his confidence and reputation within the social group (Pepler and Craig 2000). The adult responsible for supporting the victimized youth must ensure that there is no retaliatory aggression, and she/he must do this by maintaining close communication with those involved.

FORMATIVE CONSEQUENCES FOR THE CHILDREN
OR YOUTH WHO BULLY OR HARASS

An effective policy specifies the actions and formative consequences for the youths who have bullied or harassed a peer. The responses to bullying and harassment must be applied consistently, and, as with the responses to the victim, their intensity must match the severity of the alleged unwelcome behaviour. A consistent response to bullying and harassment serves several purposes: it signals support for the youth being victimized or harassed; it recognizes the need for interventions to support the individual who has been harassing; and it conveys a public message that bullying and harassment will not be tolerated within the school or organization, thereby promoting a positive and safe climate.

In all cases, students should be held responsible for their bullying or harassing behaviour. In responding, it is important not to bully the youth who has engaged in bullying as this generates feelings of hostility and alienation. We recommend establishing formative consequences that not only provide a clear message that bullying is unacceptable but that also build awareness and skills to promote students' responsibility and positive leadership (Pepler and Craig 2000). Formative consequences provide support for students to learn the skills and acquire the insights that they are lacking. In this way, the consequences for bullying can provide an opportunity to educate and support students who are in difficulty. Through formative consequences, students who bully can learn to turn their negative power and dominance into positive leadership. The policy to support aggressive youths can specify that subsequent steps be taken to garner support within other salient systems in the youth's lives, such as the family, peer group, school, and community. At no point should we give up on aggressive youths and, by denying them access to support, essentially declare them unsalvageable. If we expel the highest-risk youths from schools or community settings, we exclude them from the potential of receiving supportive interventions in a safe context. Research shows that there are effective interventions for rehabilitating even the most troubled youths of our society (Chamberlain and Reid 1998; Henggeler et al. 1998).

CONCLUSION

Peer bullying and victimization has recently been highlighted by educators, researchers, and concerned parents. There is a substantial body of research on youth aggression and victimization that provides a strong foundation from which to develop evidence-based practices and interventions. These individuals recognize that bullying and victimization pose critical obstacles to youths' healthy educational, social, and emotional adjustment. Without intervention, these youths are likely to be trapped in a snowballing pattern of negative interactions with family, teachers, peers, and romantic partners. Their possibilities for adaptive change become increasingly constrained over time as they become alienated from many essential socializing influences and supports. The high prevalence of bullying and victimization and its associated negative effects for youth represent a significant cost to our society, as measured by concurrent and long-term outcomes, as well as the lost potential of our youth. The UN Convention on the Rights of the Child identifies adults as being responsible to protect children from all forms of violence. Bullying and harassment constitute abuse at the hands of peers and violate the rights of youths. At the same time, adolescents must be involved in planning and developing programs that have the potential to be effective. The time has come for individuals, families, schools, organizations, and governments to demonstrate responsibility and leadership in addressing problems of bullying and victimization.

In implementing the principles set down in the UN document, a national initiative to raise awareness and to support both the perpetrators and victims of bullying is much needed. We have recently been funded from the Networks of Centres of Excellence New Initiative (NCE-NI) program for such an initiative, called PREVNet (Promoting Relationships and Eliminating Violence/La Promotion des Relations et l'Élimination de la Violence – www.prevnet.ca). We are able to develop a network of researchers linked to a network of national non-government organizations and government departments. Through this broad, national collaboration, PREVNet is promoting: education and training, assessment and evaluation, prevention and intervention, and policy and advocacy. The PREVNet perspective is systemic, focusing on the youths involved in bullying and victimization as well as on their peers, parents, schools, and communities. PREVNet's mission is to promote healthy relationships for all children and youths in our society, wherever they live, work, and play. Through PREVNet partnerships, we aim to protect the democratic right of children and youths to be safe and to grow up in health-promoting positive relationships with other children and youths as well as with adults. In the face of the WHO survey, in which, in the area of bullying, Canada's performance was dismal, it is essential that we, as a society, assume the responsibility of reducing violence and ensuring the health and well-being of our children. Bullying may lay the foundation for the consolidation of more violent behaviours. By preventing and addressing the problems of bullying and victimization in adolescence, we will contribute to the efforts to build a secure, equitable, and productive society.

REFERENCES

American Psychological Association (APA). 2001. *Publication Manual of the American Psychological Association*. 5th ed. Washington, DC: APA.

Atlas, R., and D.J. Pepler. 1998. Observations of bullying in the classroom. *Journal of Educational Research* 92:86–99.

Bjorkqvist, K., K. Osterman, and A. Kaukiainen. 1992. The development of direct and indirect aggressive strategies in males and females. In *Of*

Mice and Women: Aspects of Female Aggression, ed. K. Bjorkqvist and P. Niemela, 51–64. New York: Academic Press.

Boivin, M., S. Hymel, and E. Hodges. 2001. Toward a process view of peer rejection and harassment. In *Peer Harassment in School: The Plight of the Vulnerable and Victimized*, ed. J. Juvonen and S. Graham, 263–89. New York: Guilford Press.

Chamberlain, P., and J.B. Reid. 1998. Comparison of two community alternatives to incarceration for chronic juvenile offenders. *Journal of Consulting and Clinical Psychology* 6:624–33.

Connolly, J., W. Craig, A. Goldberg, and D. Pepler. 1999. Conceptions of cross-sex friendships and romantic relationships in early adolescence. *Journal of Youth and Adolescence* 28:481–94.

Connolly, J., D.J. Pepler, W.M. Craig, and A. Tardash. 2000. Dating experiences and romantic relationships of bullies in early adolescence. *Journal of Maltreatment* 5:299–310.

Craig, W.M., S. Goldbaum, M. King, and W.F. Boyce. 2001. *Health Risks and Correlates of Bullying and Victimization*.

Craig, W.M., and Y. Harel. 2004. Bullying, physical fighting, and victimization. In *Young People's Health in Context: International Report from the* HBSC *2001/02 Survey*, ed. C. Currie, C. Roberts, A. Morgan, R. Smith, W. Settertobulte, O. Samdal, and V. Barnekow Rasmussen, 133–144. WHO Policy Series: Health Policy for Children and Adolescents, Issue 4. Copenhagen: WHO Regional Office for Europe.

Craig, W.M., and D.J. Pepler. 1995. Peer processes in bullying and victimization: An observational study. *Exceptionality Education in Canada* 5:81–95.

– 1997. Observations of bullying and victimization on the school yard. *Canadian Journal of School Psychology* 13:41–60.

Craig, W.M., D.J. Pepler, and R. Atlas. 2000. Observations of bullying on the playground and in the classroom. *International Journal of School Psychology* 21:22–36.

Craig, W.M., D. Pepler, J. Connolly, and K. Henderson. 2001. Developmental context of peer harassment in early adolescence. In *Peer Harassment in School: The Plight of the Vulnerable and Victimized*, ed. J. Juvonen and S. Graham, 242–61. New York: Guilford Press.

Dishion, T.J., J. McCord, and F. Poulin. 1999. When interventions harm: Peer groups and problem behavior. *American Psychologist* 54:755–764.

Farrington, D. 1993. Understanding and preventing bullying. In *Crime and Justice*, ed. M. Tonry and N. Morris, 17:381–458. Chicago: University of Chicago Press.

Finkelhor, D., N. Assdigan, and J. Dziuba-Leatherman. 1995.
Victimization and prevention programs for children: A follow-up.
American Journal of Public Health 85:1684–989.

Ford, D.H., and R.M. Lerner. 1992. *Developmental Systems Theory:
An Integrative Approach*. Newbury Park: Sage Publications Inc.

Hawkins, D.L., D.J. Pepler, and W.M. Craig. 2001. Naturalistic
observations of peer interventions in bullying among elementary school
children. *Social Development* 10(4):512–27.

Henggeler, S.W., S.K. Schoenwald, C.M. Borduin, M.D. Rowland, and
P.B. Cunningham. 1998. *Multi-Systemic Treatment for Antisocial
Behavior in Children and Adolescents*. New York: Guilford.

Hodges, E.V.E., M. Boivin, F. Vitaro, and W.M. Bukowski. 1999. The
power of friendship: Protection against an escalating cycle of peer
victimization. *Developmental Psychology* 75:94–101.

Huesmann, L.R., L.D. Eron, M.M. Lefkowitz, and L.O. Walder. 1984.
Stability of aggression over time and generations. *Developmental
Psychology* 20:1120–34.

Juvonen, J., and S. Graham, eds. 2001. *Peer Harassment in School: The
Plight of the Vulnerable and Victimized*. New York: Guilford Press.

King, A.J.C., W.F. Boyce, and M. King. 1999. *Trends in the Health of
Canadian Youth*. Ottawa: Health Canada.

King A.J.C., B. Wold, C. Tudor-Smith, and Y. Harel, eds. 1996. *The
Health of Youth: A Cross-National Survey*. WHO Regional Publications,
European Series No. 69. Copenhagen: World Health Organization.

Leff, S.S., J.B. Kupersmidt, C.J. Patterson, and T.J. Power. 1999. Factors
influencing teacher identification of peer bullies and victims. *School
Psychology Review* 28:505–17.

Mahady-Wilton, M., W.M. Craig, and D.J. Pepler. 2000. Emotional
regulation and display in classroom bullying: Characteristic expressions of affect, coping styles and relevant contextual factors. *Social
Development* 2:226–44.

McMaster, L., J. Connolly, D.J. Pepler, and W.M. Craig. 1998. *Mental
Health Outcomes for Victims of Sexual Harassment*. Poster presented
at the biennial meetings of the Society for Research on Adolescence,
San Diego.

– 2002. Peer to peer sexual harassment among early adolescents.
Development and Psychopathology 14:95–105.

O'Connell, P., D.J. Pepler, and W.M. Craig. 1999. Peer involvement in
bullying: Insights and challenges for intervention. *Journal of
Adolescence* 22:437–52.

Olweus, D. 1991. Bully/victim problems among school children: Some basic facts and effects of a school-based intervention program. In *The Development and Treatment of Childhood Aggression*, ed. D. Pepler and K. Rubin, 411–448. Hillsdale, NJ: Erlbaum.

– 1992. Victimization by peers: Antecedents and long-term outcomes. In *Social Withdrawal, Inhibition, and Shyness in Childhood*, ed. K.H. Rubin and J.B. Asendorf, 315–341. Hillsdale, NJ: Erlbaum.

– 1993. *Bullying at School: What We Know and What We Can Do.* Oxford: Blackwell.

– 1994. Annotation: Bullying at school: Basic facts and effects of a school-based intervention program. *Journal of Child Psychology and Psychiatry and Allied Disciplines* 35(7):1171–90.

Patterson, G. R. 1986. The contribution of siblings to training for fighting: A microsocial analysis. In *Development of Antisocial and Prosocial Behavior*, ed. D. Olweus and J. Block, 235–61. New York, NY: Academic Press.

Patterson, G.R., B.D. DeBaryshe, and E. Ramsey. 1989. A developmental perspective on antisocial behaviour. *American Psychologist* 44:329–35.

Pepler, D., and W. Craig. 2000. *Making a Difference in Bullying: The LaMarsh Report.* Toronto: LaMarsh Centre for Research on Violence and Conflict Resolution, York University.

Pepler, D.J., Craig, W.M., and J. Connolly. 1997. Bullying and victimization: The problems and solutions for school-aged children. *Fact sheet for the National Crime Prevention Council of Canada.*

Pepler, D.J., W.M. Craig, J. Connolly, and A. Yuile. 2001. A developmental perspective on bullying and victimization. Manuscript in preparation.

Pepler, D., W.M. Craig, P. O'Connell, R. Atlas, and A. Charach. 2004. Making a difference in bullying: Evaluation of a systemic school-based program in Canada. In *Bullying in Schools: How Successful Can Interventions Be?*, ed. P.K. Smith, D.J. Pepler, and K. Rigby, 125–140. Cambridge: Cambridge University Press.

Pepler, D.J., W.M. Craig, S. Ziegler, and A. Charach. 1994. An evaluation of an anti-bullying intervention in Toronto schools. *Canadian Journal of Community Mental Health* 13:95–110.

Perry, D.G., E.V.E. Hodges, and S.K. Egan. 2001. Determinants of chronic victimization by peers: A review and a new model of family influence. In *Peer Harassment in School: The Plight of the Vulnerable and Victimized*, ed. J. Juvonen and S. Graham, 73–104. New York: Guilford Press.

Rigby, K. 2001. Health consequences of bullying and its prevention in schools. In *Peer Harassment in School: The Plight of the Vulnerable and Victimized,* ed. J. Juvonen and S. Graham, 310–31. New York: Guilford Press.

Schwartz, D., L.J. Proctor, and D.H. Chien. 2001. The aggressive victim of bullying: Emotional and behavioral dysregulation as a pathway to victimization by peers. In *Peer Harassment in School: The Plight of the Vulnerable and Victimized*, ed. J. Juvonen and S. Graham, 147–74. New York: Guilford Press.

Sharpe, S., and P.K. Smith, eds. 1994. *Tackling Bullying in Your School: A Practical Handbook for Teachers* London: Routledge.

Smith, P.K., H. Cowie, R.F. Olafsson, and A.P.D. Liefooghe. 2002. Definitions of bullying: A comparison of terms used, and age and gender differences, in a fourteen-country international comparison. *Child Development* 73:1119–33.

Smith, P.K., D.J. Pepler, and K. Rigby, eds. 2004. *Bullying in Schools: How Successful Can Interventions Be?* Cambridge: Cambridge University Press.

Sutton, J., P.K. Smith, and J. Swettenham. 1999. Social cognition and bullying: Social inadequacy or skilled manipulation? *British Journal of Developmental Psychology* 17:435–50.

United Nations. 1989. *Convention on the Rights of the Child.* Geneva: United Nations.

10

Injury and Youth: Scope of the Injury Problem and Implications for Policy

TREVOR L. STROME
AND LOUIS HUGO FRANCESCUTTI

INTRODUCTION

Injury is the leading cause of death and disability facing adolescents in developed countries today. In fact, injuries are the leading cause of mortality and morbidity for all people 44 years of age and under (Baker et al. 1992). The immense burden of injuries on society has been recognized by the United Nations and the World Health Organization. Three and a half million people (of all ages) worldwide die every year as the result of injuries (World Health Organization 1993). Injuries accounted for 16% of the total global burden of disease in 1998 (World Health Organization 2000).

Despite the enormity of the injury problem worldwide and despite international efforts to address injury prevention, injury remains one of the most under-recognized public health issues facing the world today. This is likely due to the fact that injuries are often viewed as "accidents" that are largely unavoidable. Injury control researchers and policy-makers, however, consider injuries to be both predictable and preventable. Policy is one of the cornerstones, along with personal responsibility, social support, and professional services, on which to build a framework that supports personal, social, environmental, and economic changes to address the injury challenge. Without policy, there would be very few (if any) product safety standards, safe and healthy workplaces, and injury prevention programs.

Adolescents' risk of being killed, permanently disabled, or severely hurt due to injury far outstrips that due to other causes such as

infectious diseases and cancer. Furthermore, the data show that
adolescents are at higher risk of injury than are other segments of
the population. It is beyond the scope of this chapter, however, to
provide an in-depth review of the many theories regarding why this
is so. Perhaps more than any other age group, adolescents face a
myriad of challenges and risk factors, ranging from peer pressure to
tumultuous physical and emotional changes that place them in harm's
way. Indeed, one of the four major principles of the United Nations
Convention on the Rights of the Child is the right to protection from
physical harm and exploitation. Article 19 of the Convention (United
Nations 1989) reads:

> 1. States Parties shall take all appropriate legislative,
> administrative, social and educational measures to protect the
> child from all forms of physical or mental violence, injury or
> abuse, neglect or negligent treatment, maltreatment or exploita-
> tion, including sexual abuse, while in the care of parent(s), legal
> guardian(s) or any other person who has the care of the child.
> 2. Such protective measures should, as appropriate, include
> effective procedures for the establishment of social programmes
> to provide necessary support for the child and for those who
> have the care of the child, as well as for other forms of preven-
> tion and for identification, reporting, referral, investigation,
> treatment and follow-up of instances of child maltreatment
> described heretofore, and, as appropriate, for judicial
> involvement.

Article 32 of the Convention reads: "1. States Parties recognize
the right of the child to be protected from economic exploitation and
from performing any work that is likely to be hazardous or to inter-
fere with the child's education, or to be harmful to the child's health
or physical, mental, spiritual, moral or social development." Policy
development is, however, particularly challenging when developing
standards, rules, and regulations for a population that needs to take
risks to test themselves and the boundaries of their environment.

The goal of this chapter is to introduce the concept of injury
control and to provide the tools that policy-makers can use to
develop, implement, and evaluate injury-related policy, especially as
it relates to adolescents. In doing so, it describes the prevalence,
seriousness, and costliness of the adolescent injury problem, illustrates

the multiple levels at which policy can be implemented, suggests which kinds of policies are most effective, and recommends how policies can affect the rate of injury occurrence. After reading this chapter, the reader will have a better understanding of the scope of the injury problem and will have the tools and understanding necessary to address the many areas in which policy can have a positive impact on the frequency of injuries in the adolescent population.

SCOPE OF THE INJURY PROBLEM AMONG ADOLESCENTS IN CANADA

Definition of Injury

An injury is any specific and identifiable bodily impairment or damage that results from an acute exposure to thermal, mechanical, electrical, or chemical energy or from the absence of essentials such as heat and oxygen (Gibson 1961). Someone breaking a leg after falling off a ladder is an example of an injury being caused by an acute exposure (the fall) to mechanical energy (hitting the ground). Similarly, a scalding burn caused by hot coffee is an example of an acute exposure to thermal energy. The word "injury" stems from the Latin word *injuria* – *in* meaning "not" and *jus* meaning "right." Literally, then, injuries are "not right."

The occurrence of injuries can be either intentional or unintentional. There are many forms of intentional injuries, which can be either self-inflicted as a result of a suicide attempt or interpersonal such as the result of violence (e.g., fist fights). There are also many examples of unintentional injuries, ranging from motor vehicle collisions and sports injuries to drowning and falls. The word "injury," unfortunately, is often associated with the word "accident." An accident is typically defined as "an unexpected and undesirable event, especially one resulting in damage or harm" (*American Heritage Dictionary of the English Language*, 4th ed., s.v. "accident"). The association of injuries and accidents implies that injuries are "freak events" that just happen, cannot be predicted, and therefore cannot be prevented. The misconception that most injuries are accidents inhibits serious examination and prevention of the possible factors and events leading to injury (Loimer, Druir, and Guarnieri 1996). However, injury researchers have shown through rigorous scientific examination that injuries are predictable, that they tend to occur in clusters (due to various factors), and, most important, that they are preventable.

Injury Statistics: Mortality, Morbidity, and PYLL

There are three major statistics used to measure and compare the absolute and relative impacts of health conditions: mortality (the number of deaths), morbidity (the number and duration of disabilities), and potential years of life lost (PYLL). PYLL is an aggregate measure commonly used in injury research that "highlights the loss to society as a result of youthful or early deaths" and is "the sum, over all persons dying from that cause, of the years that these persons would have lived had they experienced normal life expectation" (Last 1995, 128). For example, a young person dying at age 18 from an injury would result in 57 potential years of life lost, given that the individual could reasonably have been expected to live to age 75. Injuries cause more potential years of life lost than any other disease process (Baker et al. 1992).

Recent research based on data from the Health Behaviour in School-aged Children (HBSC) study suggests that the relative risk of an adolescent incurring an injury increases with the absolute number of risk behaviours engaged in by the youth, and this is reflected in both Canadian (Pickett et al. 2002) and international samples (Pickett et al., in press). Such activities include active (e.g., substance use/abuse), passive (non-use of safety gear), and independence-seeking (e.g., truancy) behaviours.

Although the actual number of injuries that occur in the general Canadian population each year is high, the rate of injury occurrences (i.e., the frequency of injuries per defined portion of the population) has been slowly decreasing. Overall, the number of injury admissions has declined by 8% in Canada from 221,313 in 1994–1995 to 204,597 in 1997–1998 (Canadian Institute for Health Information 2001). Accordingly, the rate of hospital admissions due to injury has dropped from 77 per 10,000 in 1994–1995 to 68 per 10,000 in 1997–1998. Canada can be considered middle-of-the-road in comparisons with other countries regarding injury mortality rates (Health Canada 1999b). Canada's average mortality rate due to injury between 1993 and 1995 was 44.7 per 100,000. Australia and the Netherlands fared better than Canada, with rates of 39.7 and 33.2 per 100,000 population, respectively. Scotland (49.9) and New

Zealand (55.8) fared worse than Canada. England and Wales had the lowest mortality rate at 30.5 per 100,000, whereas France had the worst at 74.7.

In North America, more children over the age of 1 year die from injuries than from cancer, heart disease, respiratory disorders, diabetes, and acquired immune deficiency syndrome (AIDS) combined (Avard and Hanvey 1989). According to Canadian injury data from the Child Injury Division, Health Protection Branch, of Health Canada (Health Canada 1999a), the leading cause of death for children aged 10 to 19 was injury. For children between the ages of 10 and 14, the mortality rate due to injury was 10.4 deaths per 100,000 population; this accounted for 52.3% of all 10- to 14-year-old deaths. For youths aged 15 to 19, the death rate due to injury was 26.1 per 100,000 population, which accounted for almost 72% of all deaths for people in that age group. Furthermore, 36.5% of all deaths to youths aged 10 to 14 were caused by unintentional injuries, and 12.8% of all deaths in that same age group were suicides. For the 15- to 19-year age group, 45.8% of all deaths were caused by unintentional injuries, whereas 22.6% of all deaths in that age group were caused by suicides.

Additional insightful information about injury morbidity in adolescents is available from Health Canada in the HBSC study from 1998. According to these data, approximately 30% to 43% (depending on grade and gender) of Canadian students were injured in 1997–1998 and required treatment by a doctor or nurse. These rates have decreased only slightly since 1994. About half of those students who required medical attention (and around 40% of those who did not) missed at least one full day of school or other activity in 1997–1998. Thus, lost academic time is a major consequence of adolescent injury.

The Canadian HBSC findings reveal that the majority of injuries occurred in the summer and fall, which correlates with times of organized sporting events that involve physical contact. The most common types of injuries suffered were strains, sprains, and pulled muscles. Bruising and internal bleeding were also common, and the occurrence of these two types of injuries tended to increase from grade 6 to grade 10.

Results indicate an interesting difference between the types of injuries suffered by girls and boys. Girls were more likely to experience sprains, strains, pulled muscles, bruising, and internal bleeding, whereas boys were more likely to have suffered broken bones, head and neck injuries, cuts, punctures, and stab wounds. For both boys and girls, there was an increase from grade 6 to grade 10 in the proportion of injuries that occurred in sports facilities and a corresponding decrease in the proportion that occurred at home.

Consequences of Injury: Economic Burden

The toll of injuries is staggering not only in terms of mortality and morbidity but also in terms of what injuries cost the health care system and society as a whole. According to Moore et al. (2001), the total economic burden of all injuries in Canada in 1998 was $12.7 billion, or 8.0% of the total Canadian burden of illness, which is estimated to be $156.9 billion. These costs include primary medical care, secondary medical supplies, time lost from school or work for both the injured person and his or her caregiver, permanent disability costs, and potential years of life lost.

The SMARTRISK Foundation (1998) estimates the annual cost of unintentional injury in Canada to be $8.7 billion. On average, each unintentional injury generates $4,000 in direct and indirect costs. Direct costs are those costs that are associated with the treatment and care of injured persons. According to SMARTRISK, unintentional injuries account for over $4.2 billion in direct costs; for example, although only about 6% of injured persons end up in hospital, hospitalization costs account for 23% of total direct costs. Indirect costs are long-term costs (such as lost wages, claims, etc.) that are associated with an injury. The estimated indirect cost of injuries is $4.5 billion. Permanent disability costs account for $2.7 billion (60%) of this amount, whereas injuries causing death account for $1.8 billion. Information regarding the monetary consequences of adolescent injury are not known, but, if PYLL is considered, these are likely to be significant.

PREVENTION AND CONTROL OF INJURIES

Haddon's Matrix

Injuries are the result of complex events in which many factors play a role. William Haddon, Jr., an engineer, physician, and well-known injury researcher, devised a tool for the logical examination of injury

Table 10.1
Haddon's Matrix for a single-vehicle motor vehicle collision

	Human factors	Agent or vehicle factors	Physical environment factors	Socio-cultural environment factors
PRE-EVENT	(1) Driver training; age; experience; alcohol; sex	(2) Design of automobile (performance, safety); quality of tires; efficiency of brakes	(3) Visibility of hazards; road curvature and gradients; divided highways; signage	(4) Social status; attitudes toward drinking and driving; graduated licensing
EVENT	(5) Utilization of safety devices (seat belt); physical fitness; resistance to injury	(6) Presence and effectiveness of safety devices (seat belt, air bag); interior design of vehicle	(7) Recovery areas; guardrails; median barriers; roadside embankments	(8) Attitudes about seat belt use; laws about seat belt use
POST-EVENT	(9) Severity of injury obtained	(10) Fire-resistance of vehicle	(11) Emergency medical services; trauma centre care; barriers to rescuing occupant	(12) Support services

events (Haddon 1972). Haddon's Matrix (10.1) is a powerful tool for debunking the "injuries are accidents" myth. The matrix serves to break down a single injury event into a series of discrete factors, each of which can increase or decrease the risk or severity of an injury. Policy-makers can utilize the matrix to identify injury-related factors and then work to eliminate or moderate factors that increase risk or severity of injury and promote or optimize factors that reduce the risk or severity of injury.

One axis of the matrix depicts three discrete time segments around the injury event: pre-event, the event itself, and post-event. The other axis of the matrix depicts various factors associated with the injury: human factors, agent or vehicle factors, physical environment factors, and socio-cultural environment factors. Human factors are the behavioural, physical, and biomechanical performance variables of the individual and include things such as fatigue, training, and overall health. Agent or vehicle factors include attributes of the mechanism and include the presence or absence of safety devices or features.

Physical environment factors are those features around the scene of an injury that contribute to its occurrence or severity. Socio-cultural environment factors include feelings, beliefs, and behaviours permeating society, or groups within society, as well as social structures in place to prevent, treat, and rehabilitate injuries.

Table 10.1 illustrates a sample Haddon's Matrix for a single-vehicle motor vehicle collision involving an adolescent driver. The pre-event row illustrates those factors and considerations that serve to either increase or decrease the chances of the motor vehicle collision occurring. Cell 1 illustrates some pre-event human factors. For example, having taken a driver's training course and one's own experience with driving can decrease the risk of collision. The use of alcohol, lack of maturity and experience, and being male, however, are other factors that can increase the risk of a motor vehicle collision. Cell 2 highlights properties of the agent or vehicle such as the design of the automobile (with respect to performance and safety), the quality of the tires (i.e., winter tires versus all-season, old tires versus new tires), and the efficiency of the brakes. Cell 3 illustrates physical environment conditions such as poor road conditions and poor weather conditions that can increase the likelihood of a collision occurring. Other factors of the physical environment include the design of the road, such as a sharp turn, steep embankment, or narrow road shoulder. Cell 4 lists socio-cultural factors that may play a role, including the social status of the driver, peer views towards driving while intoxicated, and the presence of graduated licensing programs.

The event row of Table 10.1 provides examples of factors that serve to increase or decrease the severity of an injury once the collision (the "event") has occurred. Examples of human factors at the time of the collision (Cell 5) include whether the driver is wearing a safety belt and the driver's overall physical health and resistance to injury. Vehicle factors (Cell 6) include the presence and effectiveness of safety devices (i.e., seat belt and air bag) as well as the interior design and energy-absorbing and -dissipating capability of the vehicle's frame. Properties of the physical environment (Cell 7) include surface condition of the roads, guardrails, and recovery areas. Finally, the socio-cultural environment (Cell 8) consists of evolving societal frameworks related to injury events(such as legal frameworks and industry/scientific recommendations) and public education related to prevention of such events.

The post-event row of Table 10.1 illustrates factors after the injury has occurred that can affect the outcome of the injured driver. Human factors (Cell 9) include the severity of the injury obtained and the ability of the driver to recover from the injuries. Properties of the vehicle post-event (Cell 10) that can affect the outcome of the injury include fire-resistance of the vehicle and the ease by which emergency medical rescue can extricate the driver from the vehicle. Physical and socio-cultural factors (Cells 11 and 12) include the presence of highly trained and capable emergency medical services and trauma care personnel as well as the availability of social support and rehabilitative services.

Types of Injury Prevention

The overall objective of injury-related policy is to prevent injury and therefore to reduce its impact on society in terms of both health and money. Preventing the occurrence or lessening the severity of injuries is known as primary prevention. For example, reducing the number of sports-related injuries by wearing protective gear or preventing serious bicycle-related head injuries by wearing bicycle helmets are examples of primary prevention and are largely achieved by educational and legislative/regulatory initiatives.

Secondary prevention involves the process of reducing the harmful effects of an injury once it has occurred. This normally takes the form of rapid and effective acute or trauma care that is provided as soon as possible following an injury event. Secondary prevention requires effective pre-hospital emergency medical services, highly trained acute care and trauma personnel, and up-to-date and efficient treatment facilities. High-quality and efficient secondary prevention services can reduce direct costs of injury by reducing the amount of time an individual is required to stay in hospital and by reducing unnecessary medical procedures.

Tertiary prevention facilitates the return of an individual's physical, mental, and emotional condition to her/his pre-injury status if possible. Tertiary prevention involves post-injury support such as physical and occupational therapy, workers' compensation, mental health services, and other support services. Effective tertiary prevention reduces the indirect costs of injury by minimizing an individual's time away from productive endeavours while maximizing her/his post-injury productive potential.

Primary, secondary, and tertiary prevention efforts are unlikely, independently, to have an optimal impact on reducing the occurrence and consequences of injury events. Integrating and coordinating these three prevention efforts, however, works to maximize the reduction of the occurrence and impact of injury. Such coordination between prevention efforts is known as injury control (Francescutti 1997).

Injury Control Countermeasures: Education, Environment Modification, Economics, and Enforcement

Many approaches to primary, secondary, and tertiary injury prevention are available. Each approach, however, is based on one of four basic injury control countermeasures or some combination thereof. The four major injury control strategies are: education, environment modification, economics, and enforcement. Each of these four strategies has strengths and weaknesses, and the effectiveness of each varies based on many issues, including the type and cause of injury being addressed and the population the strategy is intended to protect. Of course, each control strategy has its unique policy implications.

Education is perhaps the most common and visible injury control strategy. There are three major goals of this type of strategy: to provide information about particular injury risk and how to avoid it; to change attitudes and the way people think about injuries, their own risk of injury, and injury prevention; and to alter people's behaviours and promote empowerment for people to make decisions that reduce their injury risk.

Education is most often seen in its health promotion aspect, where people are informed of ways to reduce their risk of injury. In this role, education has taken many forms, ranging from driver's education courses to campaigns against drinking and driving. Examples of education that support primary prevention include safety campaigns that attempt to raise awareness of injuries and provide people with information about how to minimize their risk of injury. Although education efforts tend to focus on populations, they are an indispensable tool for health care providers, policy-makers, and others whose job it is to be involved in injury prevention and treatment and post-injury rehabilitation.

Education is regarded as the least effective injury control strategy since its success relies on the efforts and actions of the target audience (Christoffel and Gallagher 1999). The effectiveness of injury prevention strategies "varies inversely with the extra effort required to keep people from being harmed and the degree to which people must change their usual behaviour patterns" (Committee on Trauma Research 1985, 7). Education is, however, a very important first step. Before people can change their behaviour to reduce their risk of being injured, they must first know that injuries are a problem, that injuries are predictable and preventable, and that there are practicable measures they can take to reduce their risk of injury. Injury prevention education for adolescents, however, has the added dynamic of a natural youth interest in risk-taking for its developmental value.

Environment modification is the second major injury control strategy and encompasses efforts to reduce the likelihood of people getting into harm's way. The environments targeted by this strategy are the physical and social environments.

The physical environment encompasses the everyday surroundings of individuals that may play a role in the risk or severity of injuries. Examples of physical environmental factors include motorway design, unstable snow prone to avalanche, and the design of a playground.

The social environments include societal and behavioural factors that increase or decrease the risk or severity of injury, such as attitudes towards drinking and driving, socio-economic factors (including access to health care and financial stability), and attitudes towards wearing safety equipment or reducing risk during recreation activities.

Modifications to the physical environment are considered to be "passive" measures. They can have a positive impact on large groups of people without the specific targeting that educational programs require. Examples of physical modification include the removal (or reduction) of the potential for exposure to acute mechanical, chemical, electrical, and thermal energy that causes injuries. One example of reducing the potential energy of an injury-causing system involves the pre-emptive blasting of unstable snow to prevent an avalanche. Another way to prevent exposure to injury-causing energy is to provide a barrier between people and the source of the energy. Pedestrian overpass walkways provide a barrier between the human and the injury-causing potential energy (fast-moving traffic). Other strategies to modify the physical environment include improving highway construction and layout to minimize the risk of traffic collisions and advances in motor vehicle design (such as seat belts, improved interior design, crumple zones, and air bags).

Modifications to the social environment are not so straightforward. Improving attitudes towards injury, such as debunking the "injuries are accidents" myth, and improving the utilization rate of safety devices, such as bicycle helmets, involves different measures, including education and enforcement. Attitudes greatly affect behaviour; therefore, safety-conscious attitudes can assist with injury prevention efforts. For example, as society's acceptance of drinking and driving has gradually decreased over the years, so has the occurrence of such behaviour.

The argument behind this strategy is based on the assumption that these environments can be modified in ways that can reduce injuries. Many of the environmental factors that increase risk and severity of injuries, however, are largely human-made (e.g., motor vehicles, firearms, and poisonous chemicals). Social environment factors – such as alcohol use, attitudes conducive to risk-taking, poor social conditions, and insufficient health care – that contribute to an increased risk of injury are all more difficult to influence. Table 10.2 illustrates ten conceptual approaches, devised by Haddon, that can be utilized to modify environmental factors. The approaches illustrate how the environment can be modified by removing an injury hazard, modifying the injury hazard, protecting and modifying those at risk from the hazard, and ensuring that systems are in place to treat those suffering exposure to the hazard. It is clear that, with sufficient resources and ingenuity, the physical environment may be managed. Our ability to manage the social environment, however, has many of the same challenges as the education strategy, especially for adolescents.

Economics is a field that provides another strategy for injury prevention. Economic strategies serve to financially reward or punish individuals based on past, current, and predicted future behaviour relating to their risk of injury. One example of an economic strategy may be found in the increase of insurance premiums for individuals who have been involved in motor vehicle collisions (and the corresponding decrease for individuals not involved in motor vehicle collisions). For adolescents, economic strategies, such as high premiums for young males, may be particularly punitive due to their lower incomes and inability to earn money while in school.

Enforcement is the last major injury control strategy. Enforcement refers to the creation and application of laws and regulations with the goal of reducing the occurrence, risk, and effect of injuries.

Table 10.2
Haddon's ten conceptual approaches to injury

Approach	Example
Prevent creation of the hazard	Don't build unsafe vehicles (such as three-wheeled all-terrain vehicles)
Reduce the amount of the hazard	Package medications in smaller bottles
Prevent release of a hazard that already exists	Poison-proof a home
Modify the rate OR spatial distribution of the hazard	Install airbags in cars
Separate (in time or space) the hazard from which to be protected	Build pedestrian overpass walkways
Separate (by a material barrier) the hazard from which to be protected	Construct concrete medians between oncoming lanes of traffic
Modify basic qualities of the hazard	Build cribs with slats too narrow to strangle a child
Make what is to be protected more resistant to damage from the hazard	Ensure people are healthy and in good physical condition
Begin to counter the damage already done by the hazard	Train people to conduct first aid
Stabilize, repair, and rehabilitate the object of the damage	Integrate primary, secondary, and tertiary prevention (establish an injury control system)

Enforcement is not an end in itself and is not used as an injury control strategy in isolation; rather, it usually incorporates one or more of the other control strategies to target high-priority injury problems. Enforcement measures can be directed at individuals or groups of people by mandating or prohibiting specific behaviours and activities (see section entitled "Graduated Licensing" later in this chapter). Legislation can also be directed at commercial products by setting design and performance standards or by imposing certain restrictions. Finally, laws can be directed at environmental conditions or physical places and serve to mandate or prohibit certain conditions.

In Canada, each province and territory, as well as the Parliament of Canada, is a sovereign body granted legislative authority by the Canadian Constitution Act to enact statutes. The legislative competence of each body, however, is limited specifically to certain classes of matters (Gall 1983, 31). There are three major sources of legislation: acts, regulations, and bylaws. Acts are written laws that are formally passed by either federal or provincial governments; regulations are rules that are made under the authority of a statute by government departments or ministries that are responsible for carrying out the statute; and, finally, bylaws are written laws that are formally passed by a municipality (Gibson and Murphy 1984).

Currently, there is no concerted effort to coordinate injury legislation to ensure that there are no gaps and that the best strategies and countermeasures are being employed. There are, however, numerous injury-related laws that span various governmental jurisdictions and departments and that attempt to prevent many types of injuries through a variety of strategies. These various laws have been enacted over time without any unifying injury control strategy in mind. For example, all provinces in Canada have legislation that mandates the utilization of seat belts while travelling in motor vehicles (e.g., the national rate in Canada for seat belt use has increased from 81.4% in 1992 to 90.1% in 2000) (Transport Canada 2000). Yet, some provinces allow unbelted passengers in the payload section of pickup trucks, while others do not. HBSC data indicate that adolescent use of seat belts has decreased slightly from 66% in 1994 to 62% in 1998.

Enforcement of laws aimed at preventing injuries is effective mainly because, due to a fear of repercussions, people affected by legislation change their behaviours in accordance with the laws. The effectiveness of laws is greatest when people are apt to comply with the law independent of enforcement, if it is easy to get caught when in noncompliance, and if few exceptions to the rule are permitted.

INJURY DATA SOURCES

Policy-makers must understand injury risk factors and the effectiveness of intervention strategies in order to develop policy that alleviates those risks. Risk factors related to person, place, and time for the occurrence of injury can be determined by studying the etiology (causes) of injury events. To better understand these factors, policy-makers require accurate, timely (up-to-date), and readily available injury data. There are several sources of data that are available to be used for research and for guiding the development of injury policy. Common data sources include vital statistics, hospital records, injury surveillance systems, and trauma registries. In many provinces, the de facto standard sources for injury data are from provincial government vital statistics and hospital administrative databases. Injury mortality data are abstracted from the vital statistics database, whereas injury morbidity data are abstracted from the hospital databases.

Injury surveillance systems are an excellent source of injury data that policy-makers can utilize when making policy decisions. Epidemiologic surveillance is "the systematic collection, analysis, interpretation, and sharing of health data for the design, implementation, and evaluation of public health programs" (Langmuir 1963, 191). Comprehensive public health surveillance enhances injury research and policy development because surveillance data are disseminated in a timely manner, utilized to support and evaluate prevention and control activities, and provide ongoing monitoring of important health issues (Garrison et al. 1994). The Canadian Hospitals Injury Reporting and Prevention Program (CHIRPP) is an injury surveillance system instituted in 1990 to study the rates, etiology, and outcomes of injuries to children and youth. The primary focus of the CHIRPP system is on injuries to people 19 years of age and under. CHIRPP is a computer-based system researchers use to collect and analyze childhood and adolescent injuries and poisonings from sixteen emergency departments across Canada. CHIRRP has been cross-validated with the national HBSC database and has been determined to contain nationally representative data (Pickett et al. 2000).

Trauma registry systems, either hospital-based or representative of a health region, are another common source of injury data. Trauma registries are intended to collect trauma information from defined groups over time and "create data bases on injured patients cared for within a given institution, association, region, or governmental jurisdiction" (Rodenberg 1996, 205). Trauma registries are most often utilized by large urban trauma centres and are very often linked with an academic institution. There has been an increase in the number of trauma registries contributing injury-related information for both clinical and administrative purposes (Ehlinger, Gardber, and Nakayama 1990).

EXAMPLES OF INJURY POLICY IN ACTION

There are literally hundreds of examples of injury policy, ranging from federal government statutes and municipal bylaws to safe workplace and school safety initiatives. Some policy has proven to be effective and some has not. Following are examples of three well-publicized injury policy initiatives that affect adolescents.

Graduated Licensing

The National Highway Traffic Safety Administration (1999) estimates that teenage drivers are involved in up to three times the number of fatal motor vehicle crashes as are other drivers. This dismal statistic is due to three major factors that put this age group at much higher risk for motor vehicle collisions: inexperience, risk-taking behaviour, and risk exposure. Inexperience is not a surprising factor because they are new drivers and have not had the time to develop the skills required to handle all traffic situations. Teenage drivers are also prone to more risk-taking behaviour, whether it is to impress their friends or because they do not apprehend the likelihood of negative consequences. Young drivers are keen to get behind the wheel to take advantage of their new-found freedom; therefore, their enthusiasm for driving, which results in frequent excursions, increases their risk of exposure to situations that their limited experience is unable to handle.

Several Canadian provinces and US states have implemented graduated licensing systems for new drivers. Graduated licensing systems operate on the premise that, if you mitigate the risk factors (inexperience, risk-taking behaviour, and exposure to risk) facing new and young drivers, then it is possible to reduce the number of teenage-driver fatalities. For example, by removing a likely cause of risk-taking behaviour (such as distractions by friends in the vehicle) and preventing exposure to risky situations (such as driving at night), young novice drivers will be able to mature and to increase their driving experience in a risk-reduced environment during the graduated licensing period. Graduated licensing systems create this risk-reduced environment, which allows novice drivers to accumulate experience, safe driving practices, and safe attitudes by implementing a staged licensing process in which initial licensure restrictions (such as no driving at night and restrictions on passengers in the vehicle) are gradually lifted as the novice driver demonstrates continued improvements in skill and judgment.

Results from the Province of Ontario illustrate the positive impact of graduated licensing programs. After implementation of the graduated licensing programs in 1996, the Ontario Ministry of Transport reported that the total number of collisions involving novice drivers decreased by 31%. Similarly, the fatality rate for novice drivers dropped by 24%.

In Nova Scotia, analysis has shown that implementation of a graduated licensing program was associated with a significant reduction in overall motor vehicle collisions and casualties (Mayhew, Simpson, and des Groseilliers 2000). There was a 24% decrease in total motor vehicle collisions during the first full year of the program for drivers aged 16 years. Furthermore, a 37% reduction in crashes occurred over the first three years of the program. Interestingly, the positive results of graduated licensing are not limited to young novice drivers: after implementation of the program, there was a decrease in the collision rate by 19% for all new drivers.

Graduated licensing programs are an example of injury-related policy that has had a very positive impact on the rate and severity of injuries occurring to adolescents.

Impaired Driving

Alcohol consumption is perhaps the greatest hazard to driving. As a driver's blood alcohol concentration (BAC) increases to 0.10 (a concentration of 0.10 g or 100 mg of alcohol in 100 ml of blood), the risk of being involved in an alcohol-related motor vehicle collision gradually increases. Once the BAC crosses the 0.10 threshold, the risk of a crash actually increases exponentially with increasing amounts of alcohol consumed. Drivers whose blood alcohol concentrations lie within the range of 0.10 to 0.25 are six to thirty-two times more likely to become involved in a crash than are those drivers who have not been drinking. In the United States in 1999, 35.1% of traffic fatalities (2,238) involving people 20 years of age and under were alcohol-related. Of the alcohol-related fatalities, 74% were males (National Highway Traffic Safety Administration 1999). In Canada, 40% of teenage drivers killed and 23% of teenage drivers seriously injured in motor vehicle crashes had been drinking (Mayhew, Simpson, and des Groseilliers 2000).

The solution to impaired driving is obvious: ensure that people who have been drinking do not get behind the wheel. Some studies suggest that crashes due to impaired driving could be prevented by publicizing intensive law-enforcement efforts. Provided that the penalties are severe enough and that enforcement of impaired driving laws is effective, the prevention model suggests that the number of impaired driving crashes could be reduced by deterring potential offenders from drinking and driving.

Under the Criminal Code of Canada, it is an offence to be in control (or have care of) a motor vehicle if one's blood alcohol concentration exceeds 0.08. Police are able to charge a driver with impaired driving even if the driver's BAC is below 0.08, provided it is demonstrated that the driver's ability to operate the vehicle is impaired. Furthermore, all provinces, excluding Quebec, have legislation that empowers police to temporarily suspend for a short time period (twelve to fourteen hours) the licence of a driver whose BAC is measured to be over 0.50 (or 0.40 in Saskatchewan). Under the Criminal Code, penalties for a first offence of driving while impaired, driving with a BAC over 0.08, or refusing to provide a breath sample include a twelve- to thirty-six-month suspension from driving, a minimum $600 fine, or up to six months in jail for a summary offence or up to five years in jail for an indictment. Penalties for a third offence (or more) include a thirty-six-month to lifetime prohibition from driving, a fine of up to $2,000 if a summary offence, without maximum if an indictment, and at least ninety days in jail (up to six months if a summary offence or five years if an indictment). Strategies that help enforce drinking and driving laws include strict enforcement of impairment laws, prompt suspension of licences for people arrested for impaired driving, and sobriety checkpoints (DeJong and Hingson 1998). Enforcement can be compounded with underage alcohol consumption laws.

Fortunately, efforts to curb impaired driving appear to be working. Since the beginning of the 1980s, there has been a relatively consistent decline in the number of fatally injured drivers who tested positive for alcohol. At that time, about 60% of all drivers killed in motor vehicle crashes tested positive for alcohol. In 1997, that number had reached an all-time low of 33% (Mayhew, Beirness, and Simpson 2000), but it has since rebounded to approximately 38% in 2001 (Mayhew, Beirness, and Simpson 2004). Factors that have likely played a role in the reduced numbers of impaired drivers include: (a) campaigns that raise awareness of the dangers involved in drinking and driving, (b) stricter law enforcement, and (c) innovative prevention programs that offer alternative methods of transportation, designated drivers, and responsible practices for serving alcohol to intoxicated patrons (CDC/National Highway Traffic Safety Administration 1992; Graham 1993).

Cycling

Bicycle riding is a very common sporting and recreational activity. Bike-related injuries, however, cost Canadians $200 million every year. The majority of deaths and disabilities due to bicycle-riding result from injury to the head. Based on observational studies, it is estimated that 82% of Alberta's cyclists (19 years of age and under) who suffered a bike-related major trauma were not wearing a helmet at the time of the injury (ACICR 2000). Approximately 75% of bicyclist fatalities and about 66% of bicyclist hospital admissions were a result of head trauma (Rivara et al. 1998). Roughly 90% of all bicycle-rider fatalities due to head injuries result from a collision with a motor vehicle (Centers for Disease Control and Prevention 1995).

There are many studies that demonstrate that bicycle helmets that are worn properly and consistently are very effective in reducing the occurrence and severity of head injury. For example, studies suggest that the use of helmets while riding a bicycle can reduce the risk of a head or brain injury by 70% and can reduce injuries to the upper- or mid-face by 65% (Rivara et al. 1998). Other studies have shown that injuries to the head were much less common among bicyclists wearing a helmet than they were among those not wearing a helmet (Thompson, Rivara, and Thompson 1996; Maimaris et al. 1994).

The demonstrated effectiveness of bicycle helmets with regard to preventing and reducing the severity of head and face injuries has spurred the development of various policies to encourage (and enforce) the wearing of helmets. Laws that mandate the use of helmets have succeeded in increasing the percentage of bicyclists who wear helmets (Puder et al. 1999). Results from one Australian state (Victoria) show an increase in bicycle helmet use from 30% to 75% following enactment of the law, while the number of head injuries suffered by bicyclists decreased (Cameron et al. 1994). Following implementation of a bicycle helmet law in New Zealand, helmet use among school-aged children increased along with a corresponding decrease in the number of serious head injuries (Scuffham and Langley 1996). In 1996, British Columbia became the first Canadian province to enact a bicycle helmet law. Following implementation of the law, helmet utilization by bicyclists on commuter routes increased from 60% in 1995 to 75% in 1999. Among adolescents in Canada, however, bicycle helmet use is still low. HBSC data in 1998 indicated that the proportion of adolescents who often or always wear a helmet decreased from 57% in grade 6 to 17.5% in grade 10 (King, Boyce, and King 1999). Difficulties such as inconsistent legislation and enforcement vis-à-vis minors may be responsible for these low rates in Canada.

SUMMARY

This chapter provides policy-makers with tools to develop well-informed, evidence-based, and effective policies to address the wide-ranging challenge of adolescent injuries. Other readers who will benefit from this chapter include educators, community planners, health care professionals, and youth groups. Using tools such as Haddon's Matrix, it is possible to analyze injury events by their constituent components (human, agent or vehicle, and physical and social environment factors), permitting policy-makers to study injury occurrences and allowing examination of injuries from virtually any aspect. When seemingly "random accidents" are thoroughly analyzed, patterns and factors emerge to reveal elements not immediately obvious that can be addressed to prevent injury occurrence, reduce severity, or improve chances of successful rehabilitation.

There is an imbalance in the resources allocated to injury research and prevention. Currently, less than one cent is spent on injury prevention research and control for every dollar that is spent on treating injuries. Contrast this situation with the cancer field, where nine cents is spent on research for every dollar spent on treatment, even though the annual burden of illness due to injury is higher than that due to cancer (Moore et al. 1997). Due to the tremendous return on investment, funding for injury prevention research and control measures is money well spent. In many cases, injury prevention interventions are inexpensive and easy to implement. For example, every dollar spent on a bicycle helmet saves $30 in direct and indirect costs of injury. Every dollar that is spent on traffic check-stops to prevent drinking and driving saves $8 in injury costs. Each dollar spent on a child car seat saves up to $32 in direct and indirect costs. Finally, every dollar that is spent on a smoke detector can save $65 for the health care system and society (Centers for Disease Control and Prevention 2000). It is clear that simple measures to prevent injuries can result in substantial savings for society.

Adolescents go through tremendous social, emotional, and physical change over a short period, and safety and injury prevention are not uppermost in their minds. In fact, decisions involving dating, school, sports, and growing up are likely to outweigh decisions regarding wearing bicycle helmets and safety gear. There are many counter-measures available that can minimize exposure to risk and allow adolescents to make safe decisions without even realizing it. Programs such as "safe grads" provide safe transportation to and from desig-nated graduation party sites. Social marketing campaigns are making it "cool" to choose to not drink or to take other mood-altering substances that can impair decisions while driving, while at work, or while playing sports. Adolescents are known for their creativity in "bending" the rules and in doing things their own way. Policy-makers must utilize the tools at their disposal to understand the injury risks that face adolescents today. They must be equally cre-ative, if not more so, in implementing policies that are effective in protecting adolescents from that which presents the greatest risk of death and disability: injury.

REFERENCES

Alberta Centre for Injury Control and Research (ACICR). 2000. *Bicycle Helmets Observational Study Summary.* Edmonton: ACICR.

Avard, D., and L. Hanvey. 1989. *The Health of Canada's Children: A CICH Profile.* Ottawa: Canadian Institute of Child Health.

Baker, S.P., B. O'Neill, M.J. Ginsburg, and L. Guohua. 1992. *The Injury Fact Book.* Oxford: Oxford University Press.

Cameron, M.H., A.P. Vulcan, C.F. Finch, and S.V. Newstead. 1994. Mandatory bicycle helmet use following a decade of helmet promotion in Victoria, Australia: An evaluation. *Accident Analysis and Prevention* 26:325–37.

Canadian Institute for Health Information. 2001. *National Trauma Registry: Hospital Injury Admissions Report 1998/99.* Ottawa: Canadian Institute for Health Information.

Centers for Disease Control and Prevention (CDC). 1995. Injury-control recommendations: Bicycle helmets. *Morbidity and Mortality Weekly Report*, 17 February, 44(RR-1):1–18.
– 2000. *Working to Prevent and Control Injury in the United States: Fact Book for the Year 2000*. Atlanta: CDC.
CDC/National Highway Traffic Safety Administration. 1992. *Position Papers from the Third National Injury Control Conference: Setting the National Agenda for Injury Control in the 1990s*. Washington, DC: US Department of Health and Human Services, Public Health Service, CDC.
Christoffel, T., and S. Gallagher. 1999. *Injury Prevention and Public Health*. Gaithersburg, Maryland: Aspen Publishers.
Committee on Trauma Research. 1985. *Injury in America: A Continuing Public Health Problem*. Washington, DC: National Research Council.
DeJong, W., and R. Hingson. 1998. Strategies to reduce driving under the influence of alcohol. *Annual Review of Public Health* 19:359–78.
Ehlinger, K., M.J. Gardber, and D.K. Nakayama. 1990. The trauma registry: An administrative and clinical tool. *Topics in Health Record Management* 11(2):43.
Francescutti, L.H. 1997. Injury control: Are you accountable? *Canadian Journal of Continuing Medical Education* 9 (January):109–19.
Gall, G.L. 1983. *The Canadian Legal System*, 2nd ed. Toronto: Carswell.
Garrison, H.G., C.W. Runyan, J.E. Tintinalli, C.W. Barber, W.C. Bordley, S.W. Hargarten, D.A. Pollock, and H.B. Weiss. 1994. Emergency department surveillance: An examination of issues and a proposal for a national strategy. *Annals of Emergency Medicine* 24:849–55.
Gibson, D.L., and T.G. Murphy. 1984. *All about Law: Exploring the Canadian Legal System*. 2nd ed. Toronto: John Wiley and Sons.
Gibson, J.J. 1961. The contribution of experimental psychology to the formulation of the problem of safety: A brief for basic research. In *Behavioral Approaches to Accident Research*, 77–89. New York: Association for the Aid of Crippled Children.
Graham, J.D. 1993. Injuries from traffic crashes: Meeting the challenge. *Annual Review of Public Health* 14:515–43.
Haddon, W. 1972. A logical framework for categorizing highway safety phenomena activity. *Journal of Trauma* 12:193–207.
Health Canada. 1999a. *Canadian Injury Data*. Prepared by Child Injury Division, Bureau of Reproductive and Child Health, Laboratory Centre for Disease Control, Health Protection Branch. http://www.phac-aspc.gc.ca/injury-bles/cid98–dbc98/index.html. Retrieved 1 August 2006.

- 1999b. *Measuring Up: A Health Surveillance Update on Canadian Children and Youth*. Ottawa: Health Protection Branch, Bureau of Reproductive and Child Health, Laboratory Centre for Disease Control.

King, A.J.C., W.F. Boyce, and M.A. King. 1999. *Trends in the Health of Canadian Youth* (Rep. No. C99–980276–3). Ottawa: Health Canada.

Langmuir, A.D. 1963. The surveillance of communicable diseases of national importance. *New England Journal of Medicine* 268:182–92.

Last, J.M., ed. 1995. *A Dictionary of Epidemiology*. 3rd ed. Oxford: Oxford University Press.

Loimer, H., M. Druir, and M. Guarnieri. 1996. Accidents and acts of God: A history of terms. *American Journal of Public Health* 86(1):101–7.

Maimaris, C., C.L. Summers, C. Browning, and C.R. Palmer. 1994. Injury patterns in cyclists attending an accident and emergency department: A comparison of helmet wearers and non-wearers. *British Medical Journal* 308(6943):1537–40.

Mayhew, D.R., D.J. Beirness, and H.M. Simpson. 2000. Trends in drinking-driving fatalities in Canada: Progress continues. 15th International Conference on Alcohol, Drugs and Traffic Safety, Stockholm, 22–26 May.

- 2004. Trends in drinking-driving fatalities in Canada: Progress stalls. 17th International Conference on Alcohol, Drugs and Traffic Safety, Glasgow, 8–13 August.

Mayhew, D.R., H.M. Simpson, and M. des Groseilliers. 2000. *Impact of the Graduated Driver Licensing Program in Nova Scotia: Report from the Traffic Injury Research Foundation*. Ottawa: Traffic Injury Research Foundation.

Moore R., Y. Mao , J. Zhang, and K. Clark. 1997. *Economic Burden of Illness in Canada, 1993*. Ottawa: Laboratory Centre for Disease Control, Health Protection Branch, Health Canada.

Moore, R., E. Tsakonas, J. White, and K. White. 2001. *Economic Burden of Illness, 1998*. Ottawa: Health Canada.

National Highway Traffic Safety Administration. 1999. *Youth Fatal Crash and Alcohol Facts, 1997*. Washington: National Highway Traffic Safety Administration.

Pickett, W., R.J. Brison, S. Mackenzie, M. Garner, M. King, L. Greenberg, and W.F. Boyce. 2000. Youth injury data collected by the Canadian Hospitals Injury Reporting and Prevention Program: Do they represent the Canadian experience? *Injury Prevention* 6:9–15.

Pickett, W., M. Garner, W.F. Boyce, and M. King. 2002. Gradient in risk for youth injury associated with multiple-risk behaviours: A study of 11,329 Canadian adolescents. *Social Science and Medicine* 55(6): 1055–68.

Pickett, W., H. Schmid, W.F. Boyce, K. Simpson, P. Scheidt, J. Mazur, M. Molcho, E. Godeau, A. Azzmann, M. Overpeck, and Y. Harel. In press. Multiple risk behaviours and injury: An international study of youth in 12 countries. *Archives of Pediatrics and Adolescent Medicine*.

Puder, D.R., P. Visintainer, D. Spitzer, and D. Casal. 1999. A comparison of the effect of different bicycle helmet laws in 3 New York City suburbs. *American Journal of Public Health* 89(11):1736–8.

Rivara, F.P., D.C. Thompson, M.Q. Patterson, and R.S. Thompson. 1998. Prevention of bicycle-related injuries: Helmets, education, and legislation. *Annual Review of Public Health* 19:293–318.

Rodenberg, H. 1996. The Florida trauma system: Assessment of a statewide data base. *Injury* 27(3):205–8.

Scuffham, P.A., and J.D. Langley. Trends in cycle injury in New Zealand under voluntary helmet use. 1996. 3rd International Conference on Injury Prevention and Control, Melbourne, 18–22 February.

SMARTRISK Foundation. 1998. *The Economic Burden of Unintentional Injury in Canada*. Toronto: SMARTRISK Foundation.

Thompson, D.C., F.P. Rivara, and R.S. Thompson. 1996. Effectiveness of bicycle safety helmets in preventing head injuries: A case-control study. *Journal of the American Medical Association* 276(24):1968–73.

Transport Canada. 2000. *Results of Transport Canada's July 2000 Survey of Seat Belt Use in Canada*. TP2436, Road Safety Leaflet # RS2000–02 E, October.

United Nations. 1989. *Convention on the Rights of the Child*. Geneva: United Nations.

World Health Organization. 1993. *Handle Life with Care: Prevent Violence and Negligence*. Information Kit, World Health Day, April.

– 2000. *World Health Report 1999: Making a Difference*. Geneva: World Health Organization.

PART THREE

Policy Problems, Analysis, and Recommendations

11

Improvements to the Policy Process to Increase Use of Evidence: Research Translation Examined

WILLIAM BOYCE

POLICY ANALYSIS

The four stages of policy development described by Pless (1995) and presented in Table 1.2 of this book comprise the field of policy analysis and are based on the following assumptions: that experts trained in appropriate analytical techniques can systematically apply these to the political marketplace, can discover and measure the impact of policy on citizen's interests, can project policy consequences with some accuracy, and can affect the decisions of identifiable political clients who will use the analysis to solve social problems (Shulock 1999). Scientific researchers have traditionally participated in, or contributed to, Stages 1 and 3 of Pless's policy development model, leaving the rest to policy analysts.

Observers of policy processes everywhere agree that evidence-based arguments are virtually never applied evenly either across populations or across political interests. Social theorist Theda Skocpol observes that "one of the most important facts about the power of the state may be its unevenness across policy areas. And the most telling result, even of a far-reaching revolution or reform from above, may be the disparate transformations produced across socio-political sectors" (Skocpol 1985, 17–18). In this chapter, we examine the traditional policy environment in order to better understand how research evidence fits in and what challenges and competing interests come into play when applying the results of these scientific endeavours to policy.

RESEARCH TRANSFER

Over the past decade and a half, strong advocacy has emerged for improving the understanding of the use and transfer of research – issues that have received considerable attention in the program evaluation literature (Fetterman, Kaftarian, and Wandersman 1996; Patton 1997; Torres, Preskill, and Piontek 1996). Research transfer, or ensuring that research information is transmitted effectively to users, is generally conceded to be a weak aspect of most research projects. There is also increasing interest in research transfer among policy-makers since, from their perspective, this is the final link in the research chain. Policy-makers believe that a relatively small investment of resources in understanding and improving dissemination can bring large changes in the productivity of research activities and thus their value to the policy community. Indeed an entire stream of funding has been dedicated by the Canadian Institutes for Health Research for "knowledge translation strategies" that may help link researchers to users more effectively (Davies and Boyce 2006). Additionally, the Canadian Population Health Initiative supports research programs with an explicit, and funded, mandate to disseminate research findings in creative ways.

An opposite dynamic exists as well, however, related to the tensions between ideas, interests, and institutions described by Hall (1996) and discussed earlier in this book. This is the reluctance, or inability, of policy-makers to use research ideas and evidence, especially within an environment that acknowledges that interests and institutions also have their role to play in the policy development process.

The Academic Environment

There are numerous conditions in the academic community that contribute to low levels of research utilization in policy (Glover 1995). University research usually takes a long time to yield results, often because of conflicting institutional demands on researchers to also teach and train future researchers and to administer programs. Funding bodies contribute to this time delay by providing multi-year grants for projects that could actually be done within a more concentrated time frame. In order to be awarded peer-reviewed funding, university research is often highly critical of existing studies and needs to show a specific gap in knowledge. The scientific method itself, incorporating statistical techniques that require the researcher to prove the null hypothesis (i.e., that a new intervention is *not* effective), slows the interpretation and use of findings. Publication of research in peer-reviewed journals is also a lengthy process (a problem that might be partially solved by electronic online journals). Finally, academics often search for general laws and patterns, albeit through specific studies, rather than for immediately applicable practical findings that may hold no theoretical interest. Academics tend to focus on "ideas" (as per Hall 1996) and ideal states rather than on the messy compensation issues that underlie many redistributive policy initiatives and for which policy-makers often require research.

The Policy Environment

Similarly, there are conditions in the policy environment that limit decision makers' ability to make clear requests for research. First, rigorous research requires a clear definition of a problem and variables to be measured. However, in order to satisfy opposing political "interests" (as per Hall 1996), the objectives of government policies and programs are often loosely defined and even contradictory. Broad statements of principle are often the only basis of consensus. This consensus might break down if issues and solutions were exposed to detailed research.

Second, habits of "institutions" (again, as per Hall 1996) often ensure that decision making is rushed, leaving little time for research. Thus, policy implementation tends to precede rather than follow research. Multiple policy sectors that are responsible for advancing policy do not act quickly, nor necessarily with one voice, in identifying research needs. For example, a study conducted by a ministry of education might find that student achievement would be improved by providing better nutrition in low-income areas – a problem shared with agriculture and social welfare ministries. If the latter ministries are not involved in identifying research needs, their acceptance of the research findings may be limited. Finally, governments often have too much unsynthesized information and senior policy-makers have too little time to absorb it. Merely reducing complex research findings to broad messages, however, can nullify the validity of the research endeavour. Policy-makers often fail to grasp the nuances of research ideas to the same degree that they connect with the nuances of particular interest groups.

Researcher/User Interface

The interface between researchers and policy-makers is crucial. Havelock (1980, 12) notes: "Research is used when there is effective communication between the research generator and the research user ... [it] is not a one-way process; rather, it is a dialogue which takes place over time, which allows a full sharing of concerns on both sides, and which allows for the reshaping of the message to suit the needs, concerns, and circumstances of the receiver ... [E]ffective utilization usually requires that the user participate in the knowledge-building process at various stages." Such interaction through face-to-face contact between research generators and users is increasingly recognized as the key means by which the users can learn about the research issues that concern them (Anderson et al. 1999; Richardson, Jackson, and Sykes 1990; Pless 1995; Rossi and Freeman 1993).

In a meta-analysis of over fifty studies on research utilization, Patton (1997) states that the single most important factor is the involvement of policy and program personnel in the research process. Stakeholder involvement leads to enhanced research transfer, and yet many research projects in Canadian clinical services (Lomas 1993) and community health agencies (Anderson 1997; Cosby et al. 1996) still do not emphasize a collaborative approach.

Research Translation Defined

We define the translation of evidence broadly as the process by which the subject matter of research is identified, disseminated, and applied to improve the nature and extent of health services and policies for a given population. This definition acknowledges the integral role stakeholders should have in the transfer of research (Havelock 1980; Health Services Utilization and Research Commission 1995; Patton 1997) and is consistent with work conducted recently by experts in the adolescent health promotion field (Currie and Watson 1998). For example, the HBSC study has both a scientific development group and a policy development group to ensure that researchers and policy-makers are better linked. Similarly, the Canadian Adolescents at Risk Research Network (CAARRN) attempts to link researchers and policy-makers in health and education sectors.

Distinctions in the types of research being discussed are important if the transfer of research, and its use, are to be fully understood.

Richardson, Jackson, and Sykes (1990) identify six categories of research that are relevant to decision makers: contextual or descriptive (current information on a problem or issue), diagnostic or analytical (explanations and the understanding of cause-and-effect relationships), strategic (looking at options and assessing policy alternatives), outcome evaluation (benefits/costs of a program or service provision), developmental (examining processes of implementation of a specific program), and methodological (assessing different methods and technologies). These categories of research cover the four stages of policy development suggested by Pless (1995) and outlined in Table 1.2 of this book. While there may be some overlap in this classification, it nevertheless helps to clarify what research and utilization actually mean to various parties.

MODELS OF RESEARCH UTILIZATION

In research about the knowledge translation process itself, utilization of findings has become a key concept. Early theorists Brewer and Kakalik (1979), in the Epilogue to their book *Handicapped Children*, suggest three models for utilization of research findings: knowledge-driven, decision-driven, and interactive. These are compatible with Hall's (1996) tripartite ideas-interests-institutions model.

The knowledge-driven model assumes that good ideas will, in time, surface by virtue of their correctness, appropriateness, or timeliness. A corollary is that a researcher need only circulate research containing such good ideas to a handful of influential and powerful authorities, who, in their own time and guided by their own wisdom, will respond positively and constructively. This model involves a passive approach to policy influence, which, although once popular among researchers and policy-makers, may be wasteful of resources.

The decision-driven model suggests that even information specifically sought for a particular purpose will not necessarily be used if it does not lead to an acceptable or feasible solution. This model accepts that interests and institutions are key elements in a knowledge translation environment.

Finally, the interactive model suggests that the use of research knowledge in policy-making is unlikely to occur unless a social problem has been defined by consensus, politicized, and debated. This model identifies the need to have public, as well as political, support for research findings.

Table 11.1
Benefits of research utilization for users from the policy field

Benefits	Examples
Skill benefits	• increased ability to establish appropriate research topics • development of research skills for policy staff and building overall research capacity • developing the critical capability to use appropriate research from other geographical or organizational contexts
Political and administrative benefits	• improved information bases • informed decision making
Sector benefits	• cost reduction in the delivery of services • qualitative improvements in the process of service delivery • increased effectiveness of services and equity
Broader economic benefits	• a healthier workforce • a reduction in the number of working days lost

Source: Buxton, M., and S. Hanney. 1996. How can payback from health services research be assessed? Journal of Health Services Research 1(1):35–43.

The latter two models (decision-driven and interactive) suggest that, if studies are to have an impact, then nearly as much time, effort, and resources need to be expended in the research translation phase as in the conduct of research itself. In support of this trend, there are increasing examples of research groups assessing problems, identifying potential solutions, implementing these on a pilot basis, and evaluating health outcomes (e.g., see Boyce [2000] regarding HIV/AIDS and youth). In Chapter 8, Substance Use: Harm Reduction and the Rights of the Canadian Adolescent, Christiane Poulin illustrates this process particularly well. This multi-phased process is attractive to policy-makers because it provides them with a more complete program picture upon which to base their decisions. Although this approach does take longer for policy development, it has fewer pitfalls for government decision makers.

The general benefits of research utilization for users from the policy field include several distinct categories of payback (Buxton and Hanney 1996), and these are presented in Table 11.1.

The real direct benefits of research, however, relate to its ability to contribute to long-term ideas, understanding, and enlightenment (Richardson, Jackson, and Sykes 1990). Indeed, it is often the weight of evidence that eventually leads to change in the policy environment, as mediated through decision makers' experience, political judgment, and context (Weiss and Bucuvalas 1977).

RESEARCH DISSEMINATION OPTIONS

The utilization of research knowledge is most commonly associated with the nature and extent of dissemination activities, which traditionally encompass both research reporting and distribution. Modes of research dissemination can take many forms. As noted previously, the most effective form of dissemination appears to be personal contact between the researcher(s) and the person(s) to whom the research is directed. At the other extreme is the traditional, and highly criticized, publication of findings in peer-reviewed journals solely for academic audiences. In between lie a range of options for dissemination, such as presentations at conferences and workshops, ongoing media publicity and promotion of research, regular newsletters by research organizations to their stakeholders, development of fact sheets and data tables for various audiences, and use of the Internet to communicate research findings (Lavis et al. 2002).

A key strategy for ensuring the success of dissemination efforts involves identifying, with stakeholders, the purpose and objectives of dissemination (what you want to achieve), the target audience and sector (whom you want to influence), the style and format of dissemination (how it will look), and its evaluation (what impact it has). This strategy is being effectively used by NLSCY (HRSDC 2005) and HBSC studies (Currie and Watson 1998).

CURRENT RESEARCH UTILIZATION
IN CLINICAL, COMMUNITY,
AND POLICY SETTINGS

Until recently, there was very little examination of the extent to which health research from the academic environment was effectively utilized by decision makers (Buxton and Hanney 1996; Deykin and Haines 1996; Haines and Jones 1994). In Canada, these issues have also been discussed (Anderson 1997; Anderson et al. 1999; Fooks, Cooper, and Bhatia 1997; Goel and Naylor 1993; HSURC 1995; Lomas 1990). For the most part, discussions of the use of research have focused on the clinical community (Chalmers 1991; Lomas

1993; Deykin and Haines 1996; Funk, Tornquist, and Champagne 1995; Haines and Jones 1994). Again, greater levels of interaction among researchers, practitioners, and clinical managers have been found to improve the implementation of research findings in the clinical setting.

For example, in nursing practice, the key barriers to successful implementation of research findings include inappropriate modes of dissemination, lack of time to absorb research findings, the organizational culture, and the ability of managers and clinicians to understand research reports (Cavanagh and Tross 1996; Closs and Cheater 1994; Walsh 1997).

These problems are echoed in local community agency settings. In a study of local health and social service agencies in Kingston, Ontario, several key elements were shown to affect the transfer and use of research (Anderson et al. 1999). For example, the pace of change is so rapid in service delivery environments that agencies find it difficult to develop a coherent internal research agenda, let alone take stock of the research that is being conducted in the university environment. Further, although there is a strong desire by these agencies to have greater interaction with the academic research community, most agency directors questioned just how appropriate university-based research was to the needs of the general community.

Lack of research utilization in clinical and community settings has a parallel at the policy level. A recent Canadian study (Lavis, Ross, and Hurley 2002) examines the use of health services research in health policy-making in two provinces, Ontario and Saskatchewan. Using a detailed conceptual and operational framework to examine eight policy processes, the authors conclude that only four cases used citable research at various stages of the policy process. Paradoxically, there were examples of "well-informed" policy processes that did not use specific research findings as well as "uninformed" processes that did use research. Citable research was the major mode of influence in three of the four processes that did use research findings. In these three cases, policy-makers had direct contact with researchers, often through an advisory body on the health issue at stake. The research advice actually followed by policy-makers was limited, appropriately, to professional and technical ideas on regulatory issues rather than to policy interests and institutional requirements. The authors concluded from the four cases that larger-scale decisions, involving distributive and redistributive policies, were less likely to be influenced by research. This conclusion may, however, have been influenced by the lack of health economic studies in the study cases.

INFLUENCE OF HEALTH RESEARCH ON OTHER SECTORS

If health research has had limited influence on health policy, we should expect even less of its effect on other policy sectors, which are so important to a population-health/determinants approach. In another recent study, Lavis (2002) has shown that ideas, and research, about the non-medical social determinants of health have not had a powerful influence on either agenda setting or policy development outside the health policy sector in Canada (see Table 11.2 for a sample overview of different sectors' relationship to adolescent health). Overall, Lavis (2002, 111) notes that: "It is extremely unlikely that changes in the level and distribution of health in Canada from 1971 to 1996 can be attributed to action on the basis of ideas about non-medical determinants of health ... [W]e have no evidence that these ideas have influenced policy outside the health sector." At best, policies in other sectors appear to have been formulated using symbolic ideas about health determinants, similar to those used in rhetoric on health promotion and population health.

The case of the National Children's Agenda in Canada, although not yet studied to determine whether its development used current research findings, illuminates several positive factors in the successful influence of research on child policy development: the strength of the evidence base, the clarity of the Agenda's message through studies of effective interventions, linkage between these messages and popular rhetoric, and the existence of a broad-based coalition that supports the Agenda. Unfortunately, few of these influences appear potent in the adolescent health field at this time.

Although a variety of social, behavioural, and non-medical interventions have been shown to be effective with regard to adolescent health, a relatively minor degree of policy effort and resources have been directed to these. One dominant influence lies in the active preference on the part of the public at large for health system expenditures. The Canadian public clearly wants high-quality (and expensive) medical care for illness. The public has difficulty perceiving the value of prevention activities when resources for hospital and physician care are being cut, regardless of the long-term cost inefficiencies

Table 11.2
Examples of sectoral interests involved in adolescent health issues

Health indicators	Responsible department/ministry							
	Agriculture	Transportation	Revenue	Education	Labour	Environment	Justice	Housing & Recreation
Physical activity		Bicycle paths		Physical education	Employee health screening	Clean air campaign		Sports facilities
Nutrition and obesity	Food quality		Sales tax on junk food	School meals	Health screening			Food banks
Tobacco use	Farm subsidies		Tobacco tax	Smoke-free schools	Health screening	Clean air campaign	Tobacco sales control	No smoking areas
Substance abuse			Alcohol tax	Drug-free schools	Health screening		Safe schools Drug-free schools Early diversion programs	Drug-free facilities
Responsible sexual behaviour				Anti-bullying programs	Workplace harassment policies		Sexual offence prosecutions	After-school activities

Table 11.2 (continued)

Health indicators	Responsible department/ministry							
	Agriculture	Transportation	Revenue	Education	Labour	Environment	Justice	Housing & Recreation
Mental health				After-school activities School health promotion School nursing Crisis teams	Employee assistance programs		Safe schools	Public housing revitalization
Injury and violence		Seat belt campaign Bicycle helmet law		Safe schools After-school activities	Worksite safety programs		Early diversion programs	Public housing revitalization Recreation design
Environmental quality		Highway noise control	Gasoline tax	Asbestos removal	Worksite hazardous material programs	Lead abatement Emissions standards		
Contagious disease				School health programs Immunization	Worksite health programs			

of this standard approach to health. And to complicate matters, adolescents often do not want to change health-threatening behaviours, even when they know the risks, since these behaviours have other more important social and peer benefits. The research challenge is to discover how to minimize harm to adolescents who are intent on achieving their developmental goals. The policy challenge is to educate the public about both the limits of medical care and the advantages of non-medical interventions, and to address the obstacles that prevent adolescents from freely choosing healthy behaviours. Such obstacles include an absence of supermarkets that provide healthy foods in low-income neighbourhoods, unsafe neighbourhoods that make physical activity unlikely, and advertisements that promote unsafe alcohol and tobacco use.

THE WAY FORWARD

Lomas (1990) notes that the impact of health-related research ultimately depends on the congruence of beliefs and values among researchers and research users, all of whom have varying agendas and constraints imposed by their operational environments. In Canada, it has become apparent that research must be made more relevant to stakeholder needs and policy-maker priorities (Goel and Naylor 1993; HSURC 1995). It is also apparent that increasing attention needs to be given to evidence-based decision making (National Forum on Health 1997) and that research should be disseminated more effectively (Fooks, Cooper, and Bhatia 1997). To achieve a "culture of evidence," all key stakeholders must be involved in the determination of research and its production, dissemination, marketing, implementation, and evaluation (HSURC 1995). Several initiatives have attempted to encourage more effective transfer of health-related research (Fooks, Cooper, and Bhatia 1997; OHCEN 1994). The Ontario Health Care Evaluation Network (OHCEN), for example, was created to build research-policy partnerships, ensure relevance, improve accessibility of health services research to decision makers, and encourage application of research evidence. Although many Canadian health research organizations have identified research transfer as an essential component of their activities, there is little known about the methods these organizations use to enhance the transfer process (Fooks, Cooper, and Bhatia 1997).

Academic research is best suited to defining problems from data patterns and to providing concepts and analytic methods rather than

proposing specific solutions to policy problems. Commissioned program evaluations are much more suitable for the latter purpose as
these evaluations can involve stakeholders effectively from the start
and report findings in customized formats.

Research funders must continue to play a role in funding theoretical research as this is the work that can generate novel ideas and
technologies, which can be very powerful. The trend by research
funders to devote increasing amounts to targeted research, on
defined themes and issues, should be carefully monitored to ensure
that adequate amounts are available for innovation, in addition to
confirmatory, research.

Health Canada's own policy evaluation criteria (Colvin 2002)
provide a useful model and illustrate the relative place of research
evidence (as marked with an asterisk):

- potential for improved health outcome*
- potential for reduction in health inequalities*
- established government or ministerial authority
- established federal-provincial authority
- optimal choice of instruments: potential for improved health
  outcome relative to other interventions
- appropriate exercise of federal/Health Canada role
- appropriate involvement of partners, including prior consultation
- adequate human and other resources in place to ensure relevant
  health outcomes
- is there an evidence base that supports the specific approach/
  measure being proposed?*
- how does the proposal compare with other jurisdictions (e.g.,
  WHO, OECD)?
- potential for improved health outcome for the health issue being
  addressed relative to other health issues and activities*
- degree to which measure is an essential element in fulfilling elements
  of other priorities
- value in retaining capacity to participate constructively in related
  opportunities or necessary collaborations
- potential for bridging to future opportunities

Whether these criteria are evenly or consistently applied is unknown;
however, Coleman's view of political decision making, cited in this
book, is not optimistic (Coleman 1985; Coleman and Skogstad
1990). His view is not unique to Canada. In the international health

arena, the editor of *Social Science and Medicine*, A.B. Zwi, expresses
similar views about the role of evidence in policy-making:

The evidence based health care movement to some extent
assumes a linear model of health policy-making: appropriate
insights will be fed into complex policy processes and appropriate
solutions which reflect the best available science will be implemented. This assumption is fundamentally flawed: policy-making
is not simply evidence-driven, nor should it be. Broadening the
concept of evidence to go beyond the qualitative measurement of
effectiveness and efficiency, to include qualitative determination
of the equity, sustainability, ownership, trust and political feasibility dimensions to decision making, represents a core challenge
to current policy-making. Such analyses will not necessarily
reveal a single policy prescription, but will help determine the
most appropriate mix of policies, directed at both upstream and
downstream considerations. (Zwi and Yach 2002, 1619)

This chapter dissects the complex world of research translation
and notes that, as the conceptual framework for adolescent health
expands, so do the problems in research dissemination and utilization
by various sectors.

REFERENCES

Anderson, M. 1997. The role of research transfer in local health and
    social service organizations. Paper presented at A Theory and Practice:
    Partners in Evaluation. Annual Conference of the American Evaluation
    Association, San Diego, November.
Anderson, M., J. Cosby, W. Swan, H. Moore, and M. Broekhoven. 1999.
    The use of research in local health service agencies. *Social Science and
    Medicine* 49:1007–19.
Boyce, W.F. 2000. Supporting international health policy: The role of the
    Canadian research establishment. *Canadian Journal of Development
    Studies* 21(2):207–31.
Brewer, G.D., and J.S. Kakalik. 1979. *Handicapped Children: Strategies
    for Improving Services*. Toronto: McGraw-Hill.
Buxton, M., and S. Hanney. 1996. How can payback from health
    services research be assessed? *Journal of Health Services Research*
    1(1):35–43.

Cavanagh, S.J., and G. Tross. 1996. Utilizing research findings in nursing: Policy and practice considerations. *Journal of Advanced Nursing* 24:1083–1088.

Chalmers, I. 1991. Improving the quality and dissemination of reviews of clinical research. In *The Future of Medical Journals*, ed. S.P. Lock, 127–46. London: British Medical Journal Publishing Group.

Closs, J., and F. Cheater. 1994. Utilisation of nursing research: Culture, interest, and support. *Journal of Advanced Nursing* 19:762–73.

Coleman, William D. 1985. *Business and Politics: A Study in Collective Action.* Montreal: McGill-Queen's University Press.

Coleman, William D., and Grace D. Skogstad, eds. 1990. *Policy Communities and Public Policy in Canada: A Structural Approach.* Toronto: Copp Clark Pitman.

Colvin, Phyllis. 2002. Creating the right mix. *Health Policy Research* 1(3):24–5.

Cosby, J., M. Anderson, M. Broekhoven, and W. Swan. 1996. From the researcher to the user: Finding a path for community-based research transfer. Paper presented at the International Conference on Information and Technology and Community Health, Victoria, British Columbia.

Currie, C., and J. Watson, eds. 1998. *Translating Research Findings into Health Promotion Action: Lessons from the HBSC Study.* Edinburgh: Health Educational Board for Scotland.

Davies, D., and W.F. Boyce. 2006. The Canadian Adolescents at Risk Research Network: Research for and with Youth. In *Moving Population and Public Health Knowledge into Action: A Casebook of Knowledge Translation Stories*, ed. CIHR Institute of Population and Public Health (IPPH) Canadian Population Health Initiative (CPHI), 33–6. Ottawa: Canadian Institute of Health Research (CIHR). http://www.cihr-irsc.gc.ca/e/30739.html. Retrieved 27 July 2007.

Deykin, D., and A. Haines. 1996. Promoting the use of research findings. In *The Scientific Basis of Health Services*, ed. M. Peckham and R. Smith, 138–49. London: British Medical Journal Publishing Group.

Fetterman, D.M., S.J. Kaftarian, and A. Wandersman, eds. 1996. *Empowerment Evaluation: Knowledge and Tools for Self-Assessment and Accountability.* Thousand Oaks, CA: SAGE.

Fooks, C., J. Cooper, and V. Bhatia. 1997. Making research transfer work. Summary report from the First National Workshop on Research Transfer Issues, Methods, and Experiences, Toronto, February. Co-sponsored by the Institute for Clinical Evaluative Sciences, the Institute for Work and Health, and the Centre for Health Economics and Policy Analysis.

238 William Boyce

Funk, S.G., E.M. Tornquist, and M.T. Champagne. 1995. Barriers and facilitators of research utilization: An integrative review. *Nursing Clinics of North America* 30(3):395–407.

Glover, D. 1995. Policy researchers and policy makers: Never the twain shall meet? *IDRC Reports* October:4–8.

Goel, V., and C.D. Naylor. 1993. *Using Research and Evaluation Results in Health Services Policy-making.* Working Paper Series #17. Toronto: Institute for Clinical Evaluative Sciences.

Haines, A., and R. Jones. 1994. Implementing the findings of research. *British Medical Journal* 308:1488–92.

Hall, P.A. 1996. *Politics and Markets in the Industrialized Nations: Interests, Institutions, and Ideas in Comparative Political Economy.* Cambridge, MA: Harvard University, Center for European Studies.

Havelock, R.G. 1980. Foreword. In *Using Research in Organizations: A Guide to Successful Application*, J. Rothman (author), 11–14. Beverly Hills, CA: SAGE.

Health Services Utilization and Research Commission (HSURC). 1995. Turning research into practice: Seeking partners for a participatory approach. Discussion paper. Saskatoon, SK: HSURC.

Human Resources and Social Development Canada (HRSDC). 2005. Section 7.0: Dissemination Strategy. *National Longitudinal Survey of Children and Youth (NLSCY), October 1996.* http://www.hrsdc.gc.ca/en/cs/sp/sdc/evaluation/sp-aho36e/page11.shtml. Page updated 6 June 2005. Retrieved 27 July 2007.

Lavis, J.N. 2002. Ideas at the margin or marginalized ideas? Non-medical determinants of health in Canada. *Health Affairs* 21(2):107–12.

Lavis, J.N., D. Robertson, J.M. Woodside, C.B. McLeod, and J. Abelson. 2002. How do Canadian research organizations transfer research knowledge to decision makers? Final report to the Ontario Ministry of Health and Long-Term Care. Hamilton: McMaster University.

Lavis, J.N., S. Ross, and J. Hurley. 2002. Examining the role of health services research in public policymaking. *Milbank Quarterly* 80(1):125–54.

Lomas, J. 1990. Finding audiences, changing beliefs: The structure of research use in Canadian health policy. *Journal of Health Politics, Policy, and Law* 15(3):525–42.

– 1993. Retailing research: Increasing the role of evidence in clinical services for childbirth. *Milbank Quarterly* 71(3):439–75.

National Forum on Health. 1997. *Canada Health Action: Building on the Legacy.* Vol. 2: *Synthesis Reports and Issues Papers.* Ottawa: National Forum on Health.

Ontario Health Care Evaluation Network (OHCEN). 1994. From research to informed decision: Bridging the gap. *Making Health Services Research Relevant.* Second Annual OHCEN Symposium, November. Toronto: OHCEN.

Patton, M.Q. 1997. *Utilization-Focused Evaluation.* 3rd ed. Thousand Oaks, CA: SAGE.

Pless, I.B. 1995. *Crossing the Bridge: From Research to Child Health Policy.* Montreal: McGill.

Richardson, A., C. Jackson, and W. Sykes. 1990. *Taking Research Seriously: Means of Improving and Assessing the Use and Dissemination of Research.* London, UK: Department of Health, Social and Community Planning Research, and Her Majesty's Stationery Office (HMSO).

Rossi, P., and H.E. Freeman. 1993. *Evaluation: A Systematic Approach.* 5th ed. Newbury Park, CA: SAGE.

Shulock, N. 1999. The paradox of policy analysis: If it is not used, why do we produce so much of it? *Journal of Policy Analysis and Management* 18(2):226–44.

Skocpol, Theda. 1985. Bringing the state back in: Strategies of analysis in current research. In *Bringing the State Back In*, ed. P.B. Evans, D. Rueschmeyer, and T. Skocpol, 3–37. New York: Cambridge University Press.

Torres, R.T., H.S. Preskill, and M.E. Piontek. 1996. *Evaluation Strategies for Communicating and Reporting: Enhancing Learning in Organizations.* Thousand Oaks, CA: SAGE.

Walsh, M. 1997. How nurses perceive barriers to research implementation. *Nursing Standard* 11(29):34–9.

Weiss, C.H., and M.J. Bucuvalas. 1977. The challenge of social research to decision making. In *Using Social Research in Public Policy Making*, ed. C.H. Weiss, 213–33. Lexington, MA: Lexington Books.

Zwi, A.B., and D. Yach. 2002. International health in the 21st century: Trends and challenges. *Social Science and Medicine* 54:1615–20.

12

Improvements to Research
to Benefit Policy

WILLIAM BOYCE AND IRVING ROOTMAN

In this chapter, we look at research from two perspectives: we first discuss the obstacles in applying scientific evidence to policy; we then suggest improvements to research design and conceptualization that can enhance policy.

PROBLEMS IN APPLYING SCIENCE
TO ADOLESCENT HEALTH POLICY

Inadequate Time for Applying Evidence

Most Canadian policies that focus on adolescents tend to be unco-ordinated, problem-specific, piecemeal, non-participatory, and rarely based on the most appropriate or solid evidence. There are many reasons why this is the case. A key one is that "adolescent problems" frequently attract the attention of the media, the public, and policy-makers, often resulting in demands for immediate action. This haste makes it difficult to bring together relevant evidence in the most effective manner. It also makes it difficult to mobilize key stakeholders in a coordinated and meaningful way. Policies created in haste may respond to an immediate crisis but prove themselves ineffective in the long term because they do not (a) address the determinants responsible for the problem or (b) employ evidence regarding the most effective and available interventions.

Conflicting Goals and Competing Sectors

There is increasing evidence that risk behaviours and health-enhancing behaviours of adolescents cluster within individuals and population groups (Jessor 1991; Zaslow and Takanishi 1993). It is difficult to address one type of behaviour or problem without considering others. The broad determinants of health (see Table 1.1) and related scientific evidence cannot be realistically addressed without a coordinated approach to policy-making. It is also clear from research and experience that vastly different social and physical environments, such as schools, families, neighbourhoods, and workplaces, all play an important role in determining adolescent health (US Congress, Office of Technology Assessment 1991). Furthermore, the factors that predict adolescent health – e.g., higher social class, dominant cultural group, positive family interactions, and supportive societal structures – are the same ones that support adolescent development in general (Raphael 1996). Thus, the activities encouraged by the health sector are similar in nature to those encouraged by education, social services, recreation, and other sectors.

The jurisdictional structure of Canada complicates application of research and coordination of health policies for adolescents. This structure divides authority and responsibility between the federal and provincial governments, territories, and municipalities. This geographic and political partition – even where jurisdictions overlap – makes it difficult to achieve a coordinated response to any major problem, as indicated by the recent difficulties around housing for homeless persons. It also makes it difficult to develop long-term, science-based policies immune to partisan political competition. A sample grid of the numerous sectors typically involved at the federal, provincial, and municipal levels in policy issues affecting adolescent health are presented in Table 11.2 (chapter 11).

As might be expected, there are numerous examples of how these sectors are developing contradictory policies. For example, school policy that encourages adolescents from disadvantaged backgrounds to stay in school may be in conflict with bus services that may discontinue bus passes during periods of fiscal constraint, thereby hindering adolescents from transiting between neighbouring communities. Health policy encourages adolescents to be physically active, yet the amount of physical education time in school may be reduced due to pressures to increase literacy. Recreation policy encourages adolescents to use a skateboard park, yet skateboarding teenagers may be harassed by local police.

Isolation of policy analysts from one another compounds these problems such that those who analyze risk behaviour policy (e.g., smoking, drinking, sexual practices) rarely interact with those who analyze policy in sub-populations (e.g., people with disabilities, Aboriginals) or with those who analyze policy in health-enhancing activities (e.g., nutrition, exercise). In such an environment, it is difficult to coordinate scientific arguments that may have applicability across contexts.

To further exacerbate the problem, in addition to conflicting goals, policies, and applied evidence, different sectors may also be competing for the same stock of resources to implement programs (e.g., recreation, housing, employment, education, and health).

Problems in Research Transfer

In 1974, medical sociologist David Mechanic noted that: "Medical care or health services research, in contrast to biomedical research, has had little discernable impact on public health policy, the behaviour of health professionals, or the organization of health facilities ... There is little evidence that the initiation of policy flows directly from research findings" (Mechanic 1974, 52). Decades later, this is also a core problem in health promotion.

Several reasons for these failures have been posited. First, researchers' efforts have not been directed at producing findings that are relevant to policy problems. Second, there is an unfortunate tendency for policy-makers to use results from poorly designed studies or to misuse research information for political purposes. Third, in the public health field, we are better at generating, storing, retrieving, and transmitting data than we are at absorbing, interpreting, and using information. In other words, the practical skills of knowledge synthesis and application are lacking. Chapter 11 provides a full discussion of the research transfer problem, including models and strategies to effect change.

Impediments to Researcher Influence on Policy

While researchers in applied health topics mobilize evidence in hope of influencing the formation of policy, Frank (1988, 314) notes that "public policy is established by the public (via bureaucrats and politicians), not by scientists." There exist significant impediments to researcher influence on policy. First, many researchers are unclear about the policy implications of their research – that is, about what can be changed in the real world. In order to be applied in policy development, study results must be actively translated into ideas of use to policy-makers. Second, identifying the right audience for research findings, or knowing who has influence, is difficult because hot topics and key bureaucrats frequently shift from year to year. Third, political realities require that multiple interests and constituencies be satisfied in any given policy arena, a requirement with which researchers are often uncomfortable. Fourth, in complex fields such as developmental health, there is a demand for rigorous research that reflects the big picture and helps to provide integrated answers to health problems (Keating and Mustard 1993).

For these reasons, bringing representatives of all relevant sectors to the table for meaningful dialogue and timely action is a daunting task. The requirement to involve adolescents meaningfully in the process makes policy coordination even more challenging.

Integrated Science and Integrated Policy: Not Yet a Reality

Dr Hilary Graham of the United Kingdom, writing on the topic of research on public health inequalities, notes that: "One major problem is that intersectoral policies to tackle the determinants of health inequalities require an inter-disciplinary science of health inequalities – and this science has yet to be built. Its development turns on the integration of research on health inequalities (variations in health behaviours and outcomes) and research on social inequalities (differences in social polarization and poverty), research located in separate disciplinary fields" (Graham 2002, 2006).

Graham notes that the requirements for such integrated research analysis are: available data (measures of risk exposure and outcomes) from both fields on the same population over the same time period, development of a common language (concepts and terms) between researchers, compatible methodologies of analysis, and attention to theories at both micro and macro levels of explanation.

Thus, for reasons of urgency, jurisdiction, competition, and complexity, we have not been very successful in developing integrated, or even coordinated, adolescent health policies in Canada. The fact that other countries have been similarly unsuccessful should not give us much comfort. There are examples of integrated, comprehensive social and health policy development in communities for younger children, but whether these experiences can be translated into larger-scale models is yet to be demonstrated.

Application to Local Communities

Numerous studies have demonstrated that significant variations in policy development occur across sectors, even within a single country such as Canada (Coleman and Skogstad 1990). This is often due to tensions – reported by Nelson et al. 2000 – between two aspects of policy development: evidence-based programs and community development programs. In the implementation stage, the evidence-based practice approach stresses the importance of fidelity to a program model in order to maximize the replicability that is necessary in order to demonstrate effectiveness, whereas the community development approach emphasizes adaptation of the program model to the local context in order to maximize fit and acceptance in the real world (Blakely et al. 1987). A strong theme persists in Canadian health policy development, originating from health promotion roots, that the local public must have a role in policy planning and implementation. Research on the dissemination of innovative programs – that have been shown to be effective – has found that close adherence or fidelity to the original program model is directly related to subsequent demonstrations of success in new settings (Mayer and Davidson 2000). There are also detailed descriptions of how various health constituencies, for example persons with disabilities, have played a role in adapting policy to fit local conditions in Canada (Boyce 2001).

Researchers and policy-makers argue that there is a balance needed between fidelity to the program model and adaptation to local contexts. Rigid adherence can stifle local initiative, while adapting the program to such a degree that it no longer resembles the original evidence-based program model can lead to a program that lacks the basic program components that are important for success.

PROPOSED ADJUSTMENTS TO RESEARCH
FOCUS AND COMPREHENSIVE TREND ANALYSIS

Better Understanding of Adolescence

There are a number of immediate steps that can be taken to develop a clearer understanding of adolescence. First, analyses need to assume a life-course perspective that portrays adolescence as a stage between childhood and adulthood, not as a separate population. Second, analyses need to examine relationships between various dimensions of social inequality (SES, gender, ethnicity, disability, sexual orientation) and adolescent behavioural and psychosocial risk factors, and between these same dimensions of inequality and adolescent physical and mental health outcomes. Third, the spatial determinants of health inequality (e.g., urban-rural, regional, Aboriginal reserves) need to be examined for area health effects.

Within the study of adolescent health determinants, there are key areas of focus for longitudinal study: what are the priority, or leading, determinants? For example, in the area of adolescent smoking, leading determinants could be peer/family approval, academic achievement, or availability of cigarettes. Intervention studies can address whether there are protective determinants. For example, does availability of after-school activities and neighbourhood recreational facilities protect against the risk of smoking? Cross-sectional studies can address majority/minority problems that are less changeable. For example, do gender, ethnicity, geography, and SES influence adolescent smoking?

Behavioural choices, however influenced by the above factors, are the most prominent and direct determinants of adolescent health. Daily choices made by adolescents with respect to physical activity, diet, sex, substance use, safety, and coping strategies are all important determinants of their health. For example, coping strategies that adolescents use related to body image, or peer lifestyle patterns of increasing independence and competing time-demands, could be priority behaviours in the area of eating and dieting. Are there protective behaviours? For example, does sharing of family meals at home affect eating patterns of adolescents? Are risk behaviours linked? Are there generic patterns of risk-taking that increase overall risk?

The multiple-risk concept is increasingly used to identify clusters of risk behaviours that, individually, explain small variances in adolescent health outcomes but that, collectively, explain much more (Pickett, Boyce, et al. 2002). The total number of risks taken may be more important than which risks are taken. We must, however, be aware that, regardless of the strength of the multiple-risk phenomena, the impact on population health may be small since relatively few adolescents display such clusters (Pickett, Schmid, et al. 2002).

There are few databases, though – apart from the Health Behaviour in School-aged Children (HBSC) survey – that routinely collect these data for trend analyses or that can provide comparisons with other countries. In addition, our knowledge of the magnitude, nature, and determinants of these problems at regional and local levels is much less developed, with little evidence on which to base policies.

Finally, we seldom collect and analyze information on the assets or capacities of adolescents (although the HBSC survey does this to some extent) in order to strengthen such capacities and to develop innovative interventions. Nor do we know much about the views of adolescents regarding the issues they face, their ways of addressing these issues (i.e., that would be acceptable to them), or the role they would like to play in so doing. Without the full participation of young people in the development of policy options, the interventions chosen are unlikely to succeed or to encompass the full range of innovative solutions (Boyce 2002). Involving youth in the process would be consistent with Article 13 of the United Nations Convention on the Rights of the Child, which states that the child "shall have the right to freedom of expression" (United Nations 1989).

We also need more and better information regarding the views of school and service personnel who interact with adolescents on a day-to-day basis, of policy-makers, of the media who inform the public, and of the public itself, especially parents, who have an obvious stake in the health of their children.

Intervention Research

Significantly, we lack systematic evidence regarding the effectiveness of interventions to address the problems that face adolescents. Whatever evidence we have tends to be from other countries, such as the United States and the United Kingdom. Since we know that the effectiveness of such interventions is highly dependent on the particular context and setting in which they are applied, the use of program effectiveness evidence from other countries is of questionable utility for developing adolescent health policy in Canada.

Research on Processes of Policy Development and Implementation

Finally, we have very little evidence regarding the process of development and implementation of policies focused on adolescents. Such evidence is badly needed if we want to influence and improve policy-making relevant to adolescent health problems and their determinants.

Thus, although we do have some evidence that is useful in the development and implementation of coordinated adolescent health policies in Canada, it is still relatively limited.

REFERENCES

Blakely, C.H., J.P. Mayer, R.G. Gottschalk, N. Schmitt, W.S. Davidson, D.B. Roitman, and J.G. Emshoff. 1987. The fidelity-adaptation debate: Implications for the implementation of public sector social programs. *American Journal of Community Psychology* 15:253–68.

Boyce, W.F. 2001. Disadvantaged persons' participation in health promotion projects: Some structural dimensions. *Social Science and Medicine* 52(10):1551–64.

– 2002. Influence of health promotion bureaucracy on community participation: A Canadian case study. *Health Promotion International* 17:61–8.

Coleman, William D., and Grace D. Skogstad, eds. 1990. *Policy Communities and Public Policy in Canada: A Structural Approach.* Toronto: Copp Clark Pitman.

Frank, J.W. 1988. A public health policy and the quality of epidemiological evidence: How good is good enough? *Journal of Public Health Policy* 6(3):313–21.

Graham, H. 2002. Building an inter-disciplinary science of health inequalities: The example of lifecourse research. *Social Science and Medicine* 55:2005–16.

Jessor, R. 1991. Risk behavior in adolescence: A psychosocial framework for understanding and action. *Journal of Adolescent Health* 12:597–605.

Keating, D.P., and J.F. Mustard. 1993. Social economic factors and human development. In *Family Security in Insecure Times*, ed. D. Ross, 87–105. Ottawa: National Forum on Family Security.

Mayer, J.P., and W.S. Davidson II. 2000. Dissemination of innovation as social change. In *Handbook of Community Psychology*, ed. J. Rappaport and E. Seidman, 421–38. New York: Kluwer Academic/ Plenum Publishers.

Mechanic, D. 1974. *Politics, Medicine, and Social Science.* New York: John Wiley & Sons, Inc.

Nelson, G., J. Amio, I. Prilleltensky, and P. Nickels. 2000. Partnerships for implementing school and community prevention programs. *Journal of Educational and Psychological Consultation* 11:121–45.

Pickett, W., W.F. Boyce, M. Garner, and M. King. 2002. Gradient in risk
  for youth injury associated with multiple-risk behaviours: A study of
  11,329 young Canadians. *Social Science and Medicine* 55(5):1055–68.

Pickett, W., H. Schmid, W.F. Boyce, K. Simpson, P. Scheidt, J. Mazur,
  M. Molcho, M. King, E. Godeau, M. Overpeck, A. Aszmann,
  M. Szabo, and Y. Harel. 2002. Multiple risk behaviour and injury:
  An international analysis of young people. *Archives of Pediatrics and
  Adolescent Medicine* 156:786–93.

Raphael, D. 1996. Determinants of health of North American
  adolescents: Evolving definitions, recent findings, and proposed
  research agendas. *Journal of Adolescent Health* 19:6–16.

United Nations. *Convention on the Rights of the Child.* Geneva: UN,
  1989.

US Congress, Office of Technology Assessment. 1991. *Adolescent Health.*
  3 vols. OTA-H-466, -467, -468. Washington, DC: US Government
  Printing Office.

Zaslow, M.J., and R. Takanishi. 1993. Priorities for research on
  adolescent development. *American Psychologist* 48:185–92.

13

Application of the Convention
on the Rights of the Child
to Adolescent Health Policy

EMILY BOYCE AND WILLIAM BOYCE

PART I: COMPLEXITIES OF COMBINING
A RIGHTS-BASED APPROACH
WITH EVIDENCE-BASED POLICY-MAKING
IN ADOLESCENT HEALTH

Introduction

Rights-based approaches to policy-making are increasingly valued and applied in the Canadian context. Canada ratified the United Nations Convention on the Rights of the Child (UNCRC) (United Nations 1989) in 1991. The National Children's Agenda, and a range of policy and program measures aimed at fulfilling it, have subsequently been developed. Policy aimed at improving children's health has been a key focus of the broader effort to meet the requirements of the Convention. This chapter discusses and assesses the implications of the Convention as a framework for adolescent health policy in Canada. We argue that a rights-based approach to adolescent health holds much promise but that concerted efforts to integrate evidence-based research with Convention principles and topics, or articles, are still needed to ensure appropriate and effective policy in this area.

The chapters in this book have discussed determinants, dimensions, and potential interventions in adolescent health. Authors have demonstrated how evidence-based policy-making should consider multiple determinants of health as they affect adolescents from diverse backgrounds, circumstances, and social and community contexts.

Authors who have addressed principle-based policy-making also emphasize the active role played by adolescents in affecting their own and others' health as well as the importance of policy and programming that accounts for this participation and agency. Adolescents represent a unique population group in that they simultaneously need many of the protections and forms of care accorded to "children," while seeking or being expected to engage in various "adult" forms of independence, responsibility, and participation in social and cultural life. The importance of localized, contextualized decisions in health policy-making, based on research, cannot be overstated when thinking about this complex but often underconsidered demographic group.

The Convention on the Rights of the Child is based on a set of principles that address a range of topics (United Nations 1989). The principles and topics covered by the Convention can be seen as highly congruent with a social determinants of health perspective that accounts for the complex roles played by adolescents in health. This holds true, however, only if the Convention is interpreted holistically at all times and if the interrelation between principles and articles is given thoughtful consideration. Such an interpretation of the Convention as it relates to adolescent health could be used as a framework for research agendas in order to generate appropriately nuanced and contextualized understandings of adolescent health needs and policy priorities.

As this chapter demonstrates, however, the Convention is not structured in a way that promotes such a reading or corresponding research agenda. This drawback can contribute to underdeveloped or inadequate policy for meeting adolescent health needs. In Part 1, we begin by discussing the principles of protection, development, and participation found in the Convention and some of the tensions between them as they relate to adolescent health. We consider how the structure of the Convention – with its emphasis on protection over participation and its division of topics into separate articles – can preclude an interpretation of adolescent agency and the interconnection between determinants of health. We go on to consider three major adolescent health policy issues discussed previously in this book – violence, substance use, and health promotion. We illuminate some of the problems that may arise through policy that is based on an uncritical reading of the Convention and/or that lacks attention to what the research says on these issues.

In Part 2 of this chapter, we discuss particular policies enacted in the name of the Convention since 1991 as well as broader policy trends in the Canadian context and the implications of these for adolescent health. We also review evaluations of Canada's progress in implementing the Convention, carried out by the United Nations Committee on the Rights of the Child and other child-rights organizations. Many challenges remain in balancing the prerogative of rights-based approaches to child health policy, while remaining sensitive to the realities of adolescence as a distinct developmental stage.

Rights Principles and Rights Topics in the Convention

The Convention is the first international agreement to provide children with the full set of human rights normally accorded to adults. With built-in exceptions and numerous qualifications, the Convention nevertheless sets out a unique perspective on children as individuals with civil, political, social, cultural, and economic rights. According to UNICEF (2006), this new perspective refuses previous notions of children as the property of adults or mere objects of charity; instead, the Convention views children both as members of communities and families as well as individual human subjects with their own rights. Children are to be accorded rights and responsibilities as appropriate to their level of maturity, age, and developmental stage. Further, each right is to be understood as having equal weight, and all rights are to be interpreted as interconnected (UNICEF 2006). The language and structuring of the Convention brings up questions, however, about whether, in practice, policy development processes (including priorities, methods, and theoretical approaches decided for evidence-based research) will take this holistic view or consider the unique and complex contexts of adolescent health.

The Convention may be understood as containing three main categories of human rights (herein referred to as rights principles). Children have the right to survival and development, the right to protection from harm, and the right to participation – in the exercise of their rights and in social and cultural life. As discussed in Chapter 2, the right to participation is tied to the "evolving capacities" and "age and maturity" of the child set out in Articles 5, 12, and 14.[1] Other references to participation rights (which omit to distinguish between potential differences in their application to younger and older children) are found with regard to freedom of expression and association; access to information; social integration of children with disabilities; and engagement in cultural, recreational, and artistic activity.[2] Despite appearing in just nine of forty-one substantive articles on child rights in the Convention, the rights principle of participation is intended to be taken into consideration in the application of all other rights, as are the roles of children's age, maturity, developmental stage, and evolving capacities.

The rights principle of child protection is very consistent in the Convention, with many of its articles beginning with or including close variations on the statement: "States Parties shall take all appropriate measures to protect the child from ..." The protection of children from harm emerges as a key objective in twenty-one of the Convention articles. These articles are identified in Note 3 and variously contain explicit statements or implicit assumptions that children must be protected from harm as it is directed at them from the adult world.[3] Such a view positions children as objects requiring institutional and legislative measures to ensure their protection and not as subjects or participants who play a range of interactive roles – as victims, perpetrators, willing participants, unwilling participants, coerced yet consenting participants, decisive agents, resistors of protective measures – in the issues enumerated in Note 3. In other words, children – or for our purposes specifically adolescents – play an active, and at times confrontational, independence-seeking role that goes beyond the ideas of gradual development and protection. A nuanced interpretation of the principle of participation via evolving capacities would look at the more complex, active role that adolescents, in particular, play in harmful as well as health-promoting situations. Policy approaches to these issues must recognize this duality, otherwise programs will only address the unilateral protection of young children from harmful, adult-generated forces and fail to adequately consider adolescents' agency in their lives.

The rights principle of child development is also prevalent throughout the Convention.[4] It refers to state obligations to ensure, to the maximum extent possible, the survival and development of the child. Development is considered a holistic goal and is phrased as the child's "physical, mental, spiritual, moral and social development" (Articles 27 and 32) or "the development of the child's personality, talents, and mental and physical abilities to their fullest potential" (Article 29). This conceptualization of optimum development is, for our purposes, quite compatible with a holistic view of the multiple aspects involved in full health, which is also recognized by the WHO. The participatory role of children in their own development, however, is not made explicit. The Convention consistently talks about meeting child development objectives through top-down state provision of protection, care, and services for children, often through the channel of parents and family.

The provision or existence of social supports and programs does not, however, automatically translate into improved health and development for all children. Unless national planners consider them holistically and in their complexity, articles referring to the healthy development of the child assume that children are passive recipients of care who automatically accept whatever has been decided as being in the best interest of their development. This interpretation potentially undermines the principle that children – and again particularly adolescents – play a major participatory role in their own and others' ability or inability to develop healthfully in social, peer, school, and community environments. It also ignores the reality that adolescents make active choices about whether to accept or reject information or programs aimed at improving their health. Finally, it may be argued that these articles are based on the problematic assumption that children live in families and that programs made accessible to parents or guardians (e.g., social benefits, standard of living programs, community activities) will necessarily benefit children. Such benefits may not reach adolescents who live alone, who are homeless, who rely on their own income for survival, or who, for a variety of other reasons, do not benefit from measures aimed at the family.

The Convention's emphasis on the rights principles of development and protection brings with it the risk that the role of peer influences on health – or the various impacts that young people may have on each other's mental, physical, sexual, and emotional well-being, development, and risk for harm – will be overlooked. This is a critical issue in any discussion of adolescent health. Likewise, the focus on child protection measures and on the provision of care and services to ensure child development may draw attention away from adolescent decision making about whether and in what capacities they want to gain access to services or be subject to protections and whether they feel these services or protections are truly accessible to them. Linked to this, inadequate attention may be paid to the issue of adolescent participation in the creation of programs, institutions, and policy that can contribute to their well-being and development.

The Convention's focus on protection and development implicitly leans towards early childhood issues, which, if given undue prominence, can lead to policy that does not adequately reflect the needs or rights of adolescents.

In addition to being based on the broad rights principles of development, participation, and protection, the Convention may be read as addressing a series of salient social, political, family, and cultural issues on which children are accorded human rights. These rights topics range from violence and exploitation to standard of living to access to media and arts. For the most part, rights topics are named in separate statements or articles within the Convention, and there is little cross-referencing between them. For example, the rights accorded to children with disabilities or children of minority and indigenous groups are spelled out in their own articles, but the implications of disability and minority status are not cross-referenced in articles referring to access to health services, violence and exploitation, or access to education. Another example, of particular relevance to health planners, is the lack of reference within Article 24 (on health) to many social determinants of health.

Although Article 24 on health leaves much to be desired, many of the adolescent health issues and policy priorities addressed in preceding chapters of this book are nonetheless addressed by the Convention. Further, just as the three rights principles are supposed to be upheld and applied indivisibly to each rights topic, each rights topic is meant to be considered in light of all others. This expectation of the indivisibility of rights principles and rights topics and of the need to consider their interrelatedness in policy development does in fact coincide well with a social determinants of health perspective. In adolescent health policy, this would mean thinking about how young people's health development, health protection, and health participation influences and is influenced by the many social-structural, cultural, environmental, and biological factors named as rights topics in the Convention.

Whether this occurs in practice is of question for several reasons. The structuring of the Convention does not encourage such a reading, given the inequitable distribution of the principles of protection, participation, and development across rights topics; the lack of cross-referencing between rights topics themselves; and, generally, the lack of reference to how rights topics play out in the lives of adolescents in particular. Finally, even in the event that the Convention is interpreted holistically and for its particular relevance to the stage of adolescence, it still does not indicate what appropriate and effective adolescent health policy would look like in particular national, regional, or local contexts or as applied to different groups of adolescents. These questions are best addressed through research. As the following sections demonstrate, the development of rights-based as well as locally relevant adolescent health policy in the Canadian context poses many challenges. Considerable efforts to integrate human rights with science are still needed if we are to develop an adolescent health policy built on both rights and evidence.

Violence, Substance Use, and Health Promotion: An Integrated Analysis

This section provides an analysis of three issues of relevance to adolescent health policy in the Canadian context: violence, substance use, and health promotion. We review evidence-based research featured in previous chapters and discuss the rights topics and rights principles found in the Convention on the Rights of the Child in relation to each issue. The objective is to illuminate challenges and potential directions for the integration of research with a principled approach to adolescent health policy-making in Canada.

VIOLENCE

Violence, abuse, and sexual exploitation all figure in the Convention and are also considered determinants of adolescent health. Convention references to violence are contained in articles that emphasize how States Parties are required to take measures to protect children from abuse and neglect (Article 19); sexual exploitation (Article 34); sale, trafficking, and abduction (Article 35); cruel punishment in detention contexts (Article 37); underage recruitment to armed conflicts (Article 38); and other forms of exploitation that result in harm (Article 36). As argued earlier, these articles imply the rights of children, including adolescents, to protection from violence primarily as it may be directed at them from the adult world. Clearly, policy that meets Convention standards regarding the protection of adolescents from adult violence and abuse is necessary. It is arguable, however, that such protective measures alone are inadequate and that a more critical and thorough approach to the issue of violence in the everyday lives of adolescents is required. To do this, it is necessary to integrate an analysis of adolescents' participatory and agential roles in contexts of both violence and non-violence. It is also imperative to consider the interrelation between violence and other social, environmental, and cultural conditions related to adolescent health and development.

Chapters in this book providing results of recent research on adolescent violence include Chapter 9, Responding to Bullying and Harassment: An Issue of Rights, by Debra Pepler and Wendy Craig; and Chapter 7, Sexuality and Reproductive Health in Adolescence: Policy Implications of Early Age of Sexual Debut, by Roger S. Tonkin, Aileen Murphy, and Colleen S. Poon. In these and other chapters in this book, the authors recognize the role of physical, emotional, and sexual forms of violence in determining health outcomes, such as injury, disability, mental health problems, high-risk behaviours, eating disorders, substance abuse, and problems in sexuality and reproductive health. The authors also recognize the prevalence, manifestations, and implications of violence as being connected to problems of systemic inequality and discrimination faced by particular populations. Certain adolescents' tendencies towards violent behaviour may be viewed as one manifestation of other conditions related to poor health (physical, social, emotional) and lack of material resources, either as individuals or as members of particular families or populations. Additionally, members of disadvantaged social groups are often targets for violence because violence reinforces and is facilitated by existing power inequalities between victims and perpetrators. Violence and abuse towards adolescents is thus a reflection of existing social inequalities as well as a multifaceted and integral issue affecting all aspects of population health.

The Convention does not address peer violence, and, in the absence of considerable interpretation, it does not support an integrated analysis of young people's evolving capacities as either perpetrators or targets of violence. Policy aimed at meeting the Convention guidelines with regard to violence would not necessarily address the role of adolescents in violence against peers or in perpetuating violent atmospheres, the determinants of this violence, or the corresponding need for age-appropriate and contextually relevant measures in violence prevention, reduction, resolution, or rehabilitation. Convention articles do not suggest that, in keeping with the principle of evolving capacities, policies could promote adolescents' participation in the protection of themselves or each other from violence and exploitation, be it through school programs, community programs, or other social programs.

The impacts of systemic inequality and disadvantage on adolescent health and rights are presented in Chapter 4, Socio-Economic Status and the Health and Well-being of Youths in Canada, by Lori J. Curtis; and Chapter 6, The Health and Well-being of Aboriginal Youths in Canada, by Harriet MacMillan et al. With regard to violence, girls and all adolescents from systemically disadvantaged groups are at particular risk. Aggression and violence directed at them by peers, on the basis of their sex, race, class, disability, and sexuality, can have adverse effects on personal health and development. These same inequalities and discrimination are linked to increased likelihood of sexual exploitation and other forms of abuse by adults. The systemic relation between various forms of violence and social inequality must be considered. Convention articles on violence need to be considered in light of articles on discrimination and the special needs of children from minority groups.

The prevalence of gang-related violence in Western society and the large number of adolescents involved in the sex trade (see Article 35 and the Optional Protocol on the Sale of Children, Child Prostitution, and Child Pornography, United Nations 2000), the drug trade (Article 33), and other street work are similar issues requiring attention in policy aimed at preventing or reducing the risk of violence and harm. High-risk behaviours resulting in injury and high rates of suicide among particular adolescent groups can also be viewed in relation to the right of adolescents to avoid violence and harm (for a discussion of issues in the Aboriginal community, see Chapter 6, The Health and Well-Being of Aboriginal Youths in Canada). Gang violence, self-injurious behaviour, and suicide are not mentioned in the Convention, and the reality of an active role for adolescents with regard to sex work or the drug trade is not even hinted at.

Given these omissions, there is little impetus for policy-makers to consider how young people's involvement in these activities influences or is influenced by social, economic, and cultural conditions mentioned within other Convention articles, such as discrimination and minority status, standard of living, access to education, and access to health services. The emphasis on protection of children in the Convention may also translate into policy approaches that simplistically assume that efforts to remove adolescents from exploitative or violent lifestyles will be embraced by the adolescents they target. The notion of children's evolving capacities to make decisions about their participation in social, cultural, and economic life must be integrated in policy aimed at stemming violence related to these activities. Instead of a simplistic top-down "protection" approach, the input and participation of adolescents might be sought to ensure the design of needs-based and contextually appropriate harm and risk reduction programs.

In sum, the issue of violence in the lives of adolescents is complex and interrelated with many other issues that also affect health and well-being. A critical and holistic approach to the issue of violence and adolescence should be a priority for the health community, the human rights community, and policy-makers. Preceding chapters in this book have identified violence, abuse, exploitation, and neglect as key determinants of adolescent physical, mental, and sexual health, educational achievement, and high-risk behaviour. Likewise, the prevalence and types of adolescent violence are themselves determined by an interplay of issues affecting adolescents at the individual, familial, and social levels. Furthermore, as this discussion has shown, the Convention does contain references to many of the key issues that have been identified through evidence-based research. The combination of a rights-based perspective with scientific evidence in adolescent violence has great potential if approached from a critical standpoint that recognizes the complexity of adolescents' lives.

SUBSTANCE USE

The role of substance use as a determinant of adolescent health (e.g., in terms of injury rates, health of street youth, and health in Aboriginal communities) has figured throughout this book and is treated in depth in Chapter 8, Substance Use: Harm Reduction and the Rights of the Canadian Adolescent, by Christiane Poulin. Substance use can also be viewed as a health behaviour that is determined by other factors: many authors in preceding chapters discuss systemic issues (such as youth socio-economic status, homelessness and street life, abuse, and membership in systemically disadvantaged groups) that place adolescents at heightened risk for using and abusing substances. The issues surrounding adolescent substance use are interrelated and numerous and differ across populations and communities. Effective health policy and intervention concerning substance use requires attention to localized research and evidence of problems and needs in different communities. Policy should also reflect and reinforce the Convention rights principles of protection, development, and participation and take into account multiple rights topics (also health determinants) that interact with substance use.

Direct reference to substance use in the Convention, however, is found only in Article 33 (Drug abuse). It reads: "States Parties shall take all appropriate measures, including legislative, administrative, social and educational measures, to protect children from the illicit use of narcotic drugs and psychotropic substances ... and to prevent the use of children in the illicit production and trafficking of such substances." This article does not refer to alcohol or tobacco; its overall focus is on the protection of children from illicit drugs. It is not specified how States Parties are to protect children from using drugs, though it can be inferred that protective measures would include legal repercussions for those who engage in or promote drug use, production, or trafficking among adolescents and/or legal repercussions for adolescents who use, produce, or traffic drugs. "Social and educational measures" could involve programs to educate against drug use in general or to educate about the legal repercussions of using and/or trafficking drugs, based essentially on a punitive approach. On the other hand, it may involve education and social programs aimed at reducing the risks of drug use, from a harm reduction standpoint.

When read in isolation, Article 33 of the Convention is vague and open to a range of interpretations. Children's right to protection from drug use is partly fulfilled – from a legal standpoint – once legislation and enforcement measures are put in place to criminalize drugs. It is also clear, however, that the issue needs to be addressed through social and educational policies and programs. The remaining issues for the health community revolve around adolescents' choices concerning drug and substance use. Which adolescents choose to use substances? Which groups of adolescents are at highest risk for substance abuse? What are the negative health outcomes of substance use? What are effective interventions to reduce the number of adolescents who choose to use drugs, who are at risk of turning to drugs, or who use drugs in high-risk situations? How can policy incorporate adolescents' rights to protection from the drug world with their freedom to participate in decisions concerning their own health and lives? References to drug use in the Convention do not directly encourage such questions. Such an approach is supported, however, by careful consideration of the principle of participation in relation to a range of rights topics (or health determinants) that the research indicates are connected to substance use and that are also found in the Convention.

Articles 13, 14, and 15 of the Convention, respectively, give adolescents the right to the fundamental freedoms of expression; thought, conscience, and religion; and association. Article 5 refers to adolescents' evolving capacities to exercise their own rights with regard to all other articles in the Convention. These include the right to the highest attainable standard of health and health services (Article 24); to education directed at the development of their personality, talents, and mental and physical abilities to their fullest potential (Article 29); and to appropriate information aimed at the promotion of social, spiritual, and moral well-being and physical and mental health (Article 17). Recognition of adolescents' evolving capacities to gain access to resources on their own, to exercise their rights to health and education, and to make decisions about their own personal development and lives should be part of any adolescent health policy. From this approach, adolescents' right to participation in decision making regarding substances would be integrated into policy aimed at reducing rates of substance use and corresponding high-risk behaviours.

In her chapter, author Christiane Poulin argues that substance use is inevitable among adolescents and that harm reduction programs are therefore the most progressive and effective interventions for substance users. In fact, Canada's Drug Strategy is based on the harm reduction approach, which seeks to reduce the demand for (specifically hard) drugs, reduce drug-related mortality and morbidity, and improve the effectiveness and accessibility of substance abuse information and interventions. When it comes to hard drugs and adolescents, the Convention principle of protection, which implies abstinence, is compatible with Canada's Drug Strategy objective concerning reducing the demand for hard drugs. Purely protective measures, however, aimed at full abstinence (such as those which currently exist in most Canadian schools) are not particularly useful or effective with regard to softer drugs (which may also be legal and/or accepted among adult populations). These include tobacco, alcohol, and cannabis. In these cases, harm reduction strategies that take into account adolescents' freedom of choice and that recognize – on the basis of much research-based evidence – that abstinence is often an unattainable ideal would be more realistic. Poulin points out that, despite this evidence, harm reduction (over abstinence and punitive approaches) has yet to become an accepted approach to drug education in schools.

On the other hand, the idea that harm reduction should take precedence over abstinence and prevention programs – premised on the inevitability of adolescent substance use and their right to make their own decisions about it – is not always so straightforward. In the case of tobacco use, physicians Cynthia Callard and Neil Collishaw argue that the tobacco industry's propaganda and misinformation tactics lead to adolescent choices that are fundamentally misguided (Callard and Collishaw 2002). In other words, adolescents' rights to have access to appropriate information and education aimed at full health promotion are not being upheld as long as the tobacco industry (whose main goal is profit) plays a role in educating or informing adolescents about tobacco use. In this sense, adolescent agency in substance-use decision making cannot be seen as free or as reflecting individual freedoms until the information available is aimed at both promoting health and providing accurate information upon which adolescents can base their decisions.

Appropriate education and information, in addition to health services and programs, all play a role in adolescents' choices about whether and in what capacities they use substances. The fulfillment of adolescent rights in this area thus requires attention to what measures must be put in place in order for adolescents truly to be able to participate in informed decision making about their own health. At the same time, it must recognize that some adolescents will inevitably choose to use drugs, tobacco, or alcohol and that protective or legal measures based solely on a punitive approach will not eradicate the problem. Recognition of this reality is particularly relevant to policy-makers and educators designing tobacco, alcohol, and drug education programs in schools (most of which, at this point, are based on a punitive, pro-abstinence approach). Harm reduction, however, has been adopted in Canada's Drug Strategy, which may have positive impacts on adolescents outside their schools. Finally, programs aimed at reducing systemic problems that have been shown to be determinants of substance abuse (poverty, street life, homelessness, abuse, racism, and social inequalities in communities) must also be developed if any fundamental changes are to be made in this area.

In sum, the interrelatedness of the determinants of substance use and high-risk behaviour must be recognized in adolescent health policy, as must the right of adolescents to make informed decisions. The Convention, though positive in its approach to adolescents' rights to protection from drugs, cannot be effective without this kind of combined analysis. Effective policy development (and evaluation) in the area of adolescent substance use and abuse must integrate the principles of protection and participation found in the Convention. Through reference to other rights topics found in Convention articles, as well as the evidence-based research, policy-makers must also attend to the numerous interacting social determinants of health linked to the issue of substance use.

HEALTH PROMOTION

Adolescent health and well-being has yet to become well established as a substantive focus for health promotion policy development in Canada. There seem to be three overriding and interrelated reasons for this situation, which are variously touched on in Chapter 5, Health Promotion through School Improvement; Chapter 10, Injury and Youth: Scope of the Injury Problem and Implications for Policy; and Chapter 7, Sexuality and Reproductive Health in Adolescence: Policy Implications of Early Age of Sexual Debut.

First, the lack of research on adolescent-specific issues and needs, illustrated throughout this book, means a paucity of clearly defined problems that could otherwise lead to the development of effective policy solutions. This problem compounds itself in a cyclical way: the existing lack of awareness or data on adolescent-specific health issues contributes to the ongoing under-recognition and under-funding of adolescent health research in comparison to other population groups.

Second, and connected to this paucity of data, is the tendency for adolescent issues and needs to be "lumped in" with those of either adults or younger children. Policy and programs may seek to improve adolescent health, but this is usually a secondary focus or after-thought. Examples of adult-oriented policy that may not be particu-larly adolescent-friendly – and yet are assumed to cover adolescent needs – can include community sexual and reproductive health pro-grams, mental health programs, and harm/risk reduction programs related to substance use and to physical activities such as bicycling or driving. Similarly, adolescent issues are assumed to be covered by early childhood initiatives, such as those aimed at eliminating poverty or malnutrition within families.

Third – and as both a reason for and a result of the lack of research focus on adolescent health issues – is the fact that the human rights community has yet to critically include an adolescent rights perspective.

The Convention on the Rights of the Child does not directly assist in this problem as it is silent on certain issues (e.g., adolescent sexual orientation, sexual behaviour, reproductive capacity, high-risk behaviours, suicide). The Convention is a consensus document involving many different countries and cultures, and so perhaps this omission is not surprising. The omission of these controversial issues, however, arguably weakens the document as a comprehensive guideline for many countries. Further, the Convention principle of participation (and its related concept of children's evolving capacities) does imply that policy-makers and programmers should delineate between adolescents and younger children in terms of how certain issues affect them. Unfortunately, few clues are given on how to integrate such an analysis into the policy development process.

Convention articles that outline States Parties' obligations to promote children's healthy development, as well as their evolving capacities to participate in social and cultural life and in the exercise of rights and freedoms, make implicit and at times explicit assumptions that adolescents live in families or are parented by adult guardians. Subsequently, recommendations for health promotion that are driven by the Convention may over-emphasize education and provision of resources to parents. Examples of this include Article 24 (Health and health services), which obligates States Parties to take appropriate measures to ensure that parents and children "are informed, have access to education and are supported in the use of basic knowledge of child health and nutrition, the advantages of breast-feeding, hygiene and environmental sanitation and the prevention of accidents"; and Article 27 (Standard of living), which obligates States Parties to "assist parents and others responsible for the child to implement this right [to an adequate standard of living] and shall in case of need provide material assistance and support programmes, particularly with regard to nutrition, clothing and housing." When adolescents are taken into consideration, state interventions based on these development-focused articles could only be successful if: (a) the adolescent lived at home, and (b) the adolescent accepted parental guidance and actions intended to promote her/his health. If not, such interventions would need to address the reality of adolescents' decision making and agency concerning their own nutrition and eating behaviours as well as their capacity to choose unsafe environments and high-risk activities.

It is evident that effective implementation of health promotion programs would benefit from the critical interpretation of principles within the Convention to ensure that they apply to the issues of adolescents. Likewise, the Convention needs to be expanded to include issues of adolescent sexuality, reproductive health, high-risk behaviour, and suicide, among others, if it is to be used in Canada and other countries as a tool for policy development or evaluation in the area of adolescent health. In Chapter 5, by Anderson and Boyce, for example, the authors make the case that the Convention, in principle, can be interpreted as supporting the implementation of educational and resource initiatives based on the Comprehensive School Health (CSH) model. The CSH model is based on the strategies of instruction, support services, social support, and a healthy environment, which can be and have been successfully applied to many different health issues, such as eating patterns, body image, substance use, nutrition, physical activity, sexual and reproductive health, and different high-risk behaviours. Articles 24 and 27 of the Convention can be interpreted as supporting the use of these four strategies in school health programs. It is first necessary, however, for adolescent-specific health issues and risks to be identified as requiring attention and for research to be conducted to illuminate what the focus of each CSH strategy should be for adolescents. Finally, more inclusive and diverse approaches are required in the promotion of adolescent health – approaches that distinguish it from the issues and dynamics involved in child health. These efforts would require attention to the living situations, educational status, and risk factors associated with different groups of adolescents. These groups and their issues must be identified and corresponding programs implemented in a variety of institutions, communities, and family types in order to reach out to the broadest range of adolescents.

PART 2: CANADA'S RECORD: CANADIAN POLICY SINCE RATIFICATION OF THE CONVENTION

Has Canadian policy since ratification of the Convention reflected a balanced approach to the principles of protection, development, and participation? Has it upheld the rule of the indivisibility of rights topics? Has it, in turn, improved the health of adolescents? These are difficult questions to answer since the Convention does not provide us either with a straightforward set of objectives with regard to adolescent health or with a set of indicators, measurements, or evaluation procedures. This section reviews some major policy trends as well as specific initiatives that have been under way since the early 1990s. We provide an analysis of policy of relevance to adolescent health and discuss whether, overall, it can be said that Convention priorities are being met in the Canadian context.

The relatively vague wording of Convention articles means that states will not always have similar readings or interpretations. Interpretation of the principle of participation, which corresponds with children's evolving capacities and developmental needs, is particularly relevant to adolescent health policy. As noted in Chapter 2, the rights of children to participate in the fulfillment of their own rights according to their evolving capacities as they grow older (which, for our purposes, implies rights specific to adolescents with regard to participation) is explicitly stated just three times, in Articles 5, 12, and 14. Articles 12 through 15, respectively, provide children and adolescents the right to their views; to freedom of expression; to freedom of thought, conscience, and religion; and to freedom of association. Articles 12 through 14 emphasize the role of the state and parents in providing direction and guidance to children in the exercise of these rights, in accordance with their age and maturity. The articles are vague in their outlining of fundamental freedoms, and it is unclear at what point or age adolescents can begin to be seen as free agents in the fulfillment of these rights. The challenge for decision makers is to address both the principle of evolving capacities for adolescents to participate in decisions that affect them as well as the complexity of issues facing the adolescent age group and their corresponding developmental needs.

An illustration of these tensions may be found in the case of the Canada Prenatal Nutrition Program (CPNP). It was initiated under the National Children's Agenda, itself launched as part of Canada's response to the Convention. The CPNP is a national, community-based health promotion intervention that supports community groups in creating and delivering services to pregnant, low-income, at-risk women. Its objective is to improve early childhood development in Canada. It has adopted a reflexive and participatory approach to program evaluation, which involves stakeholders in developing evaluation indicators and survey instruments with the goal of continuous program improvement (Schwendt 2002). This policy is a good example of Health Canada's evolving approach of using evidence-based research and a rights-based approach to early childhood development policy.

In another light, the CPNP can also be seen as an example of health policy that does not take into full account the needs and rights of adolescents. The goal of the CPNP is to improve birth outcomes, and its two key indicators of population impact are breastfeeding initiation rate and low birth weight rate (Schwendt 2002). The fact that 38% of the women targeted are themselves teenagers (including 9% who are 16 years old and under) (Health Canada 2005) does not emerge as a policy focus, nor do their specific needs as young, often poor, single mothers. This might be partly attributed to the fact that the Convention – and health policy based on this framework – has neglected the specific rights and needs of adolescents. In particular, the participation of adolescents in sex, reproductive matters, or childrearing is conspicuously absent in the Convention.

A stronger focus on adolescent participation in the CPNP might have led to the creation of policy whose central objective is ensuring young women's rights to have access to resources in order to make healthy decisions during pregnancy and motherhood. Similarly, an adolescent health focus might tackle underlying structural conditions that affect young mothers and influence their health (i.e., unemployment, poverty, lack of nutritious food or health resources, lack of adolescent-oriented sexual and reproductive health programs). Key indicators of program success might be based on young women's access to information and resources and their levels of empowerment as young mothers. Instead, the focus of the CPNP is on providing short-term aid to young women in order to ensure the successful gestation, birth, and early nutrition habits of their children. Overall, the CPNP is an example of much-needed, evidence-based policy whose purpose is the fulfillment of young children's rights to survival, protection, and development. It is also, however, an instance of recent policy development and evaluation that does not adequately consider the principle of participation or issues of specific relevance to adolescents.

Since ratification of the Convention in 1991, the Canadian government has developed several children's agendas or action plans to support the development of new policies. The National Children's

Agenda was launched in 1997 and contains an emphasis on early childhood development and on investing in the early years in order to improve health and well-being further down the line. The Agenda also reflects the commitment of the federal, provincial, and territorial governments to foster the health and development of adolescents. Economic security of families and fulfillment of basic needs of adolescents and younger children are considered key elements in maximizing their well-being (Federal/Provincial/Territorial Council on Social Policy Renewal 1999) and represent a recognition of the role of poverty and structural disadvantage in determining population health outcomes. On this basis, then, it also becomes arguable that, in the past fifteen years, we have witnessed a decrease or regression in Canada's efforts to improve the health of adolescents. Explanations for this unfavourable policy change include restructuring measures and cutbacks to social, health, and educational programs that would otherwise help mediate the effects of adolescent poverty and disadvantage.

Distributive assistance policies that may have benefitted adolescents and younger children in the recent past have included the addition of maternal benefits to Unemployment Insurance (UI) in 1990; the Canada Child Tax Benefit (CCTB) in 1993; the Earned Income Supplement (EIS) for low-income families with children in 1993; and the National Child Benefit Supplement (NCBS) in 1998 (which replaced the EIS and gave benefits to poor families regardless of income source). In 2000, the duration of parental leave through the Employment Insurance (EI) program was extended from six months to one year and this included paternal leave and adoptive leave. In 2000, the federal government also announced plans to add $2.5 billion to the CCTB by 2004 and to increase the disability tax credit up to $500 for families caring for a child with a disability at home. These measures were intended to counter the problem of child poverty and arguably reflect an awareness of how child poverty is often linked to the financial problems and structural barriers faced by single parents (most often mothers).

Health Canada's community programs for children, like many of the above-stated measures, also reflect a focus on improving childhood development in structurally disadvantaged and poor families. These initiatives are referred to by Health Canada (2005) as their department's contribution to the National Children's Agenda. The Community Action Program for Children (CAPC) provides long-term funding to community groups to establish and deliver services that respond to the developmental needs of children from birth to 6 years of age who are living in conditions of risk. CAPC is for children who live in low-income families, who live in teenaged-parent families, who are abused or neglected, or who are at risk of or are experiencing developmental delays. The CPNP, discussed above, provides resources to community-based groups to offer food supplements, nutrition counselling, social support, education, and referrals on lifestyle issues to pregnant women most at risk of poor birth outcomes. The Aboriginal Head Start (AHS) is an early intervention program for First Nations, Inuit, and Métis preschool children. AHS projects generally provide half-day preschool experiences to prepare young children for their school years. Finally, the Canadian Perinatal Surveillance System (CPSS) has been put in place to monitor trends and disparities on various aspects of low-income infants' health.

Most of these federal policies and community health programs for children have been aimed at low-income families and represent welcome supports to many. These initiatives may, however, be over-emphasized by the federal government as, in themselves, evidence of success rather than being accompanied by evidence regarding how they combat child poverty or improve child health and well-being. It must be remembered that these initiatives have been accompanied by massive cutbacks and reforms at the provincial level – in social assistance, mother's allowance, women's shelters, community social programs, health-care programs, subsidized housing, junior kindergarten programs, after-school programs, and subsidized child-care programs. Provincial cutbacks have been motivated, in many cases, by policies of fiscal restraint and structural changes at the federal level. For example, the federal government restricted its cost-sharing of social assistance programs with provincial governments under the Canada Assistance Plan (CAP) in 1990, putting limits on future payment increases to provinces. By 1996, CAP was replaced by the Canada Health and Social Transfer (CHST). Under this policy, the federal government began paying out block sums to provinces for health, education, and social welfare services. These sums were quantifiably less than what was previously paid out by the federal government, and provinces were given more leeway to decide how the money should be distributed across services.

Adolescent poverty has increased in recent years and may be partially attributed to fiscally conservative federal policy and continuing federal-provincial stand-offs over who provides what, and how much, for the people. In this context, the overall economic well-being of young children in Canada – let alone adolescents – has not improved. The Canadian Council on Social Development (2006) reports that the child poverty rate (of people under 18 years of age) was 15.1% in 1989. This had risen to 23.6% by 1996, and in 2003 it stood at 17.6%. In urban areas, poverty rates have been pronounced, with a recent study showing that 26% of all children aged 0 to 5, 23% of all youth aged 6 to 14, and 24% of all persons aged 15 to 24 lived in poverty (Lee 2000). Poverty is a major determinant of poor health and low educational attainment; as a result, it provides a striking indicator of the well-being of Canadian adolescents.

There have, however, been some encouraging developments in Canadian health and social research in the past fifteen years. These initiatives represent an opportunity to acquire new and more in-depth information about adolescent health and reflect progress in Canada's efforts to listen to adolescent voices and recognize them as expert informants on their own lives and health issues. Use of adolescent-informed research in policy-making can help fulfill the right of adolescents to actively participate in decision making and the policy process. For example, the National Longitudinal Survey of Children and Youth (NLSCY) was first released in 1996 and will continue as a population-based, long-term survey. It follows individuals from birth to adulthood and focuses on major aspects of well-being, including health, family, community, education, and work (HRDC and Statistics Canada 1996). The Health Behaviour in School-aged Children (HBSC) survey, however, is the first of its kind to offer information on health, health behaviours, and the family and school environments of adolescents aged 11, 13, and 15 – in Canada and in thirty-four other countries (King, Boyce, and King 1999). The particular value of the HBSC is the self-report from adolescents and its comparability with data from other similar countries.

The federal government also announced in the 2000 budget that it would allocate $20 million over a five-year period to the new Centres of Excellence for Children's Well-being. As part of the National Children's Agenda, five Centres of Excellence have been created to undertake research, respectively, in the areas of child welfare, child and youth-centred Prairie communities, early childhood development, children and adolescents with special needs, and youth engagement in health decision making. The stated goal of the centres is to collect and disseminate advanced knowledge on children's well-being to families, community organizations, educators, health professionals, and policy-makers. It will be interesting to see how this initiative contributes to a better and more complete understanding of adolescent health and what effect it has on policy-making. It should be noted, however, that the adolescence portion of the HBSC study and the Centres of Excellence (only three of which look at adolescence) are receiving only a fraction of the funding being put towards programs for early childhood development, such as CAPC and CPNP.

On all these counts, it can be said that federal policy initiated in the name of the Convention has yet to show a demonstrable effect in improving the health of adolescents. It should be noted that adolescent health has not been formed as a major focus of the National Children's Agenda. Adolescents living in low-income families may have benefitted to the same degree as young children through income supplements like the CCTB and the NCBS. Likewise, adolescents with children may have benefitted from Health Canada community programs, even if some, as teenaged parents, were not the prime targets. Canadian child health policy in the past decade and a half has not, however, reflected a substantive focus on adolescent issues or needs. Broader social, health, and education policy trends may have in fact contributed to conditions of structural disadvantage that can negatively affect adolescent health.

Reports on Canada's Progress in Implementing the Convention

Formal evaluations of Canada's success in implementing the United Nations Convention on the Rights of the Child have also indicated the inadequacy of policy initiatives intended to fit the Convention framework. The federalist system, jurisdictional disputes over funding and program responsibilities, and the lack of comprehensive data on the differing situations of Canada's adolescents and younger children combine to result in insubstantial and often inappropriate policy for meeting the real needs of these constituencies. The United Nations Committee on the Rights of the Child, the Canadian Coalition for the Rights of Children, and the International Save the Children Alliance have all highlighted the need to integrate more research data with a human rights framework in order to develop effective interventions and policy.

Canada submitted its first self-report on the Convention to the United Nations in 1994 (Government of Canada 1994), and the United Nations Committee on the Rights of the Child (1995) made several concluding observations. These observations included concern about: child poverty and a lack of programs for education, housing, and nutrition; lack of fundamental rights for vulnerable children, especially Aboriginal children, including access to housing and education; an increasing rate of adolescent suicide; restrictions in adolescents' and younger children's exercise of their fundamental freedoms of opinion in judicial and administrative hearings; jurisdictional issues and disputes contributing to disparities in child rights across the country; and the lack of a permanent monitoring mechanism to ensure children's rights at all jurisdictional levels.

The UN Committee recommended that, among other objectives, Canada create a more effective system of data collection to ensure effective federal monitoring of child rights and assessment of jurisdictional compliance with the Convention. It also recommended that Canada establish better legal and administrative coordination across jurisdictions to reduce disparities in children's rights across the country. The UN Committee did not, however, point to the need for effective data collection and analysis in order to inform and plan the development of good, localized policy; rather, it just pointed to the need to monitor policy in terms of the principles set forth in the Convention.

The Canadian Coalition for the Rights of Children (1999) submitted a non-governmental report (*The UN Convention on the Rights of the Child: How Does Canada Measure Up?*) to accompany the Government of Canada's second Convention progress report in 2001 (Government of Canada 2001). The Coalition researched six areas related to Convention articles: education, fundamental freedoms, abuse and neglect, refugee children, children with disabilities, and Canada's international obligations. In each of these areas, the Coalition found that there was a severe lack of national information and research about children under provincial and territorial authority and that this led to constraints on the development of effective policy and services. It argued that Canada needed a standardized and comprehensive system of data collection regarding children, including adolescents, at all levels of government that could be comparable over time and across jurisdictions. This data collection system was seen to be key in monitoring children's rights and in determining necessary interventions and strategies.

The International Save the Children Alliance (ISCA), which also publishes country reports, evaluations, and recommendations, has urged Canada to increase national and local spending to combat poverty; to put forth sustainable efforts towards the systemic inclusion of minority groups; to make specific efforts to improve the situation of Aboriginal youth; and to restore national standards for health care, child care, and family services (Muscroft 2000). The ISCA has focused more on the specific situation of Canadian adolescents than either the UN Committee or the Canadian Coalition on the Rights of the Child. Its report discusses the issues of adolescent sex trade workers, adolescents in the juvenile justice system, and adolescents in at-risk families and the tension that can arise between the principle of child protection and the right of children, including adolescents, to participate in decisions affecting their lives. It strongly recommends that the Canadian federal government take more responsibility for establishing a forum for increased interprovincial and interterritorial dialogue on these issues. It suggests that the federal government spend more on research activities such as the NLSCY and on research that listens to the voices of adolescents and assesses the underlying social conditions and determinants of issues affecting adolescents. This research, in turn, can be used to inform policy-making that truly ensures the rights of adolescents (Muscroft 1999).

Conclusion

Our analysis of the Convention as an over-arching framework for policy development and monitoring reveals some significant gaps in the case of adolescents. In the Convention, the rights principles of protection and development predominate over that of participation. The role of the state – often vis-à-vis support to families or adult guardians – to protect children and to provide them with care in a top-down manner is emphasized. The structuring and wording of the Convention may encourage some assumptions on the part of policy-makers that do not always hold true if we consider what the research has to say about adolescent health and needs. These include the assumptions: (a) that adolescents live in families or have guardians; (b) that families and guardians have adolescents' best interests in mind or have information about how to meet their interests; (c) that adolescents are innocent, passive recipients of the care and protection offered by families and states; (d) that adolescents will not resist protective measures and will accept what is decided as being in their best interest; and (e) that adolescents will accept others' definitions of their evolving capacities in the exercise of rights and with regard to the nature and bounds of their participation in social and cultural life. As demonstrated by our discussions of substance use, violence, and health promotion, these assumptions do not reflect the reality of adolescents' agency and participatory roles in affecting circumstances of their own and others' lives and health. Health policies and programs, if guided by Convention principles alone and without adequate interpretation, are unlikely to take into full account the needs of Canadian adolescents.

Evaluations of Canada's performance vis-à-vis the Convention illuminate many areas for improvement in the fulfillment of Convention priorities and principles. These reports consistently underscore the importance of integrating research in policy development and evaluation processes. On its own, the Convention is undoubtedly a useful tool for researchers, advocates, and policymakers with regard to conceptualizing and addressing the human rights of children. This framework is particularly important for ensuring that human rights standards are met in policy affecting adolescents. Beyond setting general standards, however, it is key that the rights topics named in various Convention articles be continuously and reflexively considered in light of all others. Like the rights principles of participation, development, and protection, the specific rights topics addressed by the Convention are supposed to be interpreted as indivisible, interconnected, and of equal importance. As such, the Convention can be seen as a framework that supports the imperative for research on adolescent health protection, development, and participation from a social determinants of health perspective. Much work remains to be done to integrate evidence-based research with Convention principles and priorities so as to ensure appropriate and effective policy in this area.

NOTES

1 Articles referring to evolving capacities/maturity level of the child:
Article 5 (Evolving capacities to exercise rights)
Article 12 (Respect for the views of the child)
Article 14 (Freedom of thought, conscience and religion)

2 Articles reflecting the principle of participation:
   Article 5 (Evolving capacities to exercise rights)
   Article 12 (Respect for the views of the child)
   Article 13 (Freedom of expression)
   Article 14 (Freedom of thought, conscience, and religion)
   Article 15 (Freedom of association)
   Article 17 (Access to information and mass media)
   Article 23 (Social integration of disabled children)
   Article 30 (Right to participate in minority culture, religion, and language)
   Article 31 (Right to cultural, leisure, artistic, and recreational activity)
3 Articles reflecting the principle of protection:
   Article 2 (Protection from discrimination and punishment)
   Article 3 (Care and protection to ensure best interests of the child)
   Article 7 (Right to name and nationality)
   Article 8 (Preservation of identity)
   Article 9 (Separation from parents)
   Article 11 (Illicit transfer and non-return of children abroad)
   Article 16 (Privacy)
   Article 17 (Protection from injurious information and media)
   Article 19 (Protection from all forms of violence)
   Article 20 (Protections for children without family)
   Article 21 (Adoption)
   Article 22 (Refugee children)
   Article 25 (Review of the treatment of children who are placed in care)
   Article 32 (Child labour)
   Article 33 (Drug Abuse)
   Article 34 (Sexual exploitation)
   Article 35 (Sale, trafficking, and abduction)
   Article 36 (Other forms of exploitation)
   Article 37 (Detention, punishment, and torture)
   Article 39 (Rehabilitation of child victims of abuse, neglect, and exploitation)
   Article 40 (Treatment by justice system)
4 Articles reflecting the principle of development:
   Article 3 (Care and protection to ensure best interests of the child)
   Article 6 (Survival and Development)
   Article 17 (Access to information and media that promotes well-being)
   Article 18 (Parental responsibility/state assistance in child development)

Article 20 (Provision of care for children without families)
Article 23 (Care for disabled children)
Article 24 (Health and health services)
Article 25 (Review of the treatment of children who are placed in care)
Article 26 (Social security)
Article 27 (Adequate standard of living)
Article 28 (Education)
Article 29 (Aims of education)
Article 31 (Provision of leisure, play, and cultural activities)
Article 39 (Rehabilitation of child victims of abuse, neglect, and exploitation)

REFERENCES

Callard, Cynthia, and Neil Collishaw. 2002. Preventing adolescent smoking through tobacco industry control. Unpublished article.

Canadian Coalition for the Rights of Children (CCRC). 1999. *The UN Convention on the Rights of the Child: How Does Canada Measure Up?* Ottawa: CCRC. http://www.rightsofchildren.ca/report/index.htm. Retrieved 28 September 2006.

Canadian Council on Social Development. 2006. *The Progress of Canada's Children and Youth.* Ottawa: CCSD. http://www.ccsd.ca/pccy/2006/economic.htm. Retrieved 8 January 2007.

Federal/Provincial/Territorial Council on Social Policy Renewal. 1999. *Developing a Shared Vision.* Ottawa: Government of Canada. http://socialunion.gc.ca/nca/may7-back_e.html. Retrieved 8 January 2007.

Government of Canada. 1994. *Canada's First Report on the Convention on the Rights of the Child.* Submitted to the United Nations, 17 June 1994. Ottawa: Heritage Canada. http://www.pch.gc.ca/progs/pdp-hrp/docs/crc/index_e.cfm. Retrieved 8 January 2007.

– 2001. *Canada's Second Report on the Convention on the Rights of the Child.* Submitted to the United Nations, 26 April 2001. Ottawa: Heritage Canada. http://www.pch.gc.ca/progs/pdp-hrp/docs/crc-2001/index_e.cfm. Retrieved 8 January 2007.

Health Canada. 2005. *Budget 2000 Information. The National Children's Agenda: Health Canada's Contribution.* Ottawa: Health Canada. http://www.hc-sc.gc.ca/ahc-asc/performance/budget/children-enfants_e.html. Retrieved 8 January 2007.

Human Resources Development Canada (HRDC) and Statistics Canada.
    1996. *Growing Up in Canada: National Longitudinal Survey of
    Children and Youth*. Ottawa: Statistics Canada.
King, Alan J.C., William F. Boyce, and Matthew A. King. 1999. *Trends
    in the Health of Canadian Youth*. Ottawa: Health Canada.
Lee, Kevin. 2000. *Urban Poverty in Canada: A Statistical Profile*.
    Ottawa: Canadian Council on Social Development (CCSD).
Muscroft, Sarah, ed. 1999. *Children's Rights: Reality or Rhetoric?
    The UN Convention on the Rights of the Child – The First Ten Years*.
    London: ISCA.
– 2000. *Children's Rights: Equal Rights? Diversity, Difference and the
    Issue of Discrimination*. London: International Save the Children
    Alliance (ISCA).
Schwendt, Steven. 2002. A Tale of Two Evaluations: CAPC and CPNP.
    Health Policy Research Bulletin March:14–18.
United Nations (UN). 1989. *Convention on the Rights of the Child*.
    Geneva, Switzerland: UN.
– 2000. *Optional Protocol to the Convention on the Rights of the Child
    on the Sale of Children, Child Prostitution, and Child Pornography*.
    Geneva: UN.
United Nations Children's Fund (UNICEF). 2006. *Convention on the
    Rights of the Child: Protecting and Realizing Child Rights*. New York:
    UNICEF. http://www.unicef.org/crc/index_30166.html. Retrieved
    22 December 2006.
United Nations Committee on the Rights of the Child. 1995.
    *Consideration of Reports Submitted by States Parties under Article 44
    of the Convention: Concluding Observations of the Committee on the
    Rights of the Child (Ninth Session): Canada*. Ottawa: Heritage
    Canada. http://www.pch.gc.ca/progs/pdp-hrp/docs/crc/crcconc_e.cfm.
    Retrieved 28 September 2006.

14

Recommendations for Developing Adolescent Health Policy

WILLIAM BOYCE

This book advocates the coordination of population-health science, rights, and policy in order to improve adolescent health and well-being. It attempts to use the United Nations Convention on the Rights of the Child as a standard for adolescent health policy development, but it also suggests that the Convention undergo critical analysis and interpretation in order to reflect the reality of adolescents. In addition, it recommends that research in the area of adolescent health and well-being, which reflects the multiple and interrelated determinants of adolescent health, needs to be conducted and disseminated on a larger scale and with attention to differences between adolescents.

In this final chapter we have a number of purposes: first, we summarize the context of evidence and human rights that underlies the policy environment; second, we explore various purposes in integrating these streams; third, we make recommendations regarding the development and coordination of adolescent health policy initiatives that both consider the changing nature of adolescent needs and encourage the involvement of civic society and adolescents themselves in policy formulation; and, finally, we note some challenges to these recommendations.

SCIENTIFIC EVIDENCE AND HUMAN RIGHTS AS A BASIS FOR POLICY-MAKING

Evidence-based decision making and the mechanisms employed to encourage uptake by policy-makers are situated within a large context. Due to structural differences in working conditions and

pressures from other sources, the link between decision makers at a
senior political level and researchers is difficult at best. Steps to
encourage interactions have not worked well. Instead of decision
makers becoming more inclined to use evidence-based policy, researchers are becoming politicized and responsive to targetted funding
initiatives. Two problems may explain this. First, policy-makers are
engaging in ad hoc decision making and temporary solutions for
good political reasons but without sound scientific grounding.
Second, universities and researchers are in a crisis of relevance as
governments cut back funding and market forces fill the gap to set
the research agenda.

The issue of adolescent health and well-being has not been a
substantive focus of the UN Convention on the Rights of the Child.
Similarly, reports on Canada's successes and failures in implementing
the Convention have neglected this issue. One of the key constraints
on most human rights conventions is their failure to address their
subjects' responsibilities, as distinct from their rights. The Convention
properly addresses the responsibilities of parents and other authorities towards children, but, as we have seen in our discussion of
adolescent health, the principle of youth responsibility is central to
the appropriate interpretation and application of the Convention.
Unfortunately, the document is silent on the responsibilities that
adolescents have by virtue of their almost-adult status. An unresolved
problem for the Convention is how its principles of protection and
promotion accommodate different theoretical models of adolescent
development – additive (simultaneous change) or predictive (trajectory) – that challenge its coherence as a unified framework for policy
planning.

THE GOAL OF COMBINING EVIDENCE
AND HUMAN RIGHTS FOR POLICY

The various relationships between scientific evidence and abstract
principles are yet to be determined. Does production of evidence
(initiated by intuition, chance, or theory) lead to development of
sound principles? Or does adherence to principles lead to research
efforts that document credible evidence of causation? It is likely that
both occur. Nonetheless, there are choices to be made in combining
science, policy, and human rights. Are we interested in coordinating
human rights policies across sectors, for example, such that adolescent

protection as a principle is achieved in education, health, justice, labour, and other sectors? If so, then we need to increase coordination between these sectors and to use common definitions and measures of the principle of protection.

Alternatively, are we interested in integrating evidence-based policies across the various domains grouped within the health sector (e.g., genetics, social/physical environment, behavioural patterns, health care) such that optimal adolescent development is addressed in each of these domains? If so, then understanding the complex interactions of determinant factors originating from these domains is essential. Is there a unifying theoretical stance, such as psychosocial development or life-course development? Or is there a diversity of conflicting stances pitting biomedical science against social inequality approaches?

Should the overall policy strategy be to develop an adolescent health agenda or to include adolescents in a public health agenda? The former strategy subscribes to Convention principles of protection and development, while the latter strategy subscribes to Convention principles of participation and equity with other groups. Are these two approaches reconcilable within a principled framework for policy?

If we are interested in combining science, policy, and human rights, then we need to simultaneously address the inconsistencies and similarities between these values and practices. Adolescent development patterns may not lend themselves easily to holistic approaches. For example, the optimal healthy life profile is one of rapid attainment and maintenance of health, peaking in the adolescent years, with increasing attention to preventing problems as one ages: this leads first to protective and then, later, to preventive health policy strategies. The optimal education profile, however, is one of more gradual attainment of knowledge and skills, peaking in middle-to-later adulthood, with more attention to lifelong learning over the life course: this leads to health-promotive strategies in education. One opportunity that these distinct sectoral profiles allow is the pursuit of cross-cutting policy impacts (such as the use of mass public education and a focus on active learning in the education system to achieve healthy living goals). One problem to be aware of, however, is that differing human development patterns in health, education, and productive work may result in unforeseen policy consequences. For example, assuming that the problems of adolescent health can

Table 14.1
Three-level policy model

Location	Policy elements	Key actors
Local	experiences and values	community members
National, regional	fusion of ideas, interests, and institutions	policy-makers
International	generalizable evidence universal principles	experts theorists

always be addressed later on may miss potential critical periods for optimizing lifelong health that occur in adolescence (e.g., delaying smoking onset in adolescents).

Finally, as mentioned numerous times in the text, what is the role of adolescents in applying localized "evidence" (or experiences from their own communities) and their particular "values" (or hopes and ideals) in the development of policy and programs?

A possible policy model drawing these local, national, and international elements together is shown in Table 14.1.

RECOMMENDATIONS

With these problems in mind, what is the way forward? The strongest allies for prevention should be adolescents themselves. Many adolescents, however, are pessimistic about their futures, relative to their parents' generation, within a global economy. Some lack the motivation to care for themselves or for others. In this context, health promotion may be viewed by adolescents as providing second-order benefits, such as longevity and increased quality of life in the long term, rather than material and career gains now. Nonetheless, adolescents are interested in the participation message of health promotion, and it may be this component that draws them into its other benefits. Thus, meaningful participation in health policy decision making may compensate for the inability of health promotion to deliver immediately on the economic and occupational goals of adolescents.

With adolescent participation, the key elements of policy change can occur. As a first step, leadership must inform and educate the public about the health promotion perspective and the commercial or professional interests and forces that threaten it. Such leadership must be multidisciplinary and able to appreciate a range of health domains and influences. In Canada, leadership could come from the minister of health or from a new secretary of state for adolescents. The Childhood and Youth Division of Health Canada is a natural leadership focus, particularly regarding education of policymakers and interest groups. The Division has already articulated a report on adolescent health, *Healthy Development of Children and Youth* (Health Canada 1999), that can provide a focus for discussion if properly disseminated. Training grounds for adolescents to become such leaders would be new interdisciplinary schools of public and human health. A new generation of leaders could emerge from such training.

Second, a range of incentives should be built into policy initiatives. These include: economic incentives and disincentives; information interventions to combat misleading advertising and media; direct regulation; indirect regulation through the court systems; and de-normalization of harmful social conditions, physical environments, and behaviours. Many of these incentives have been discussed by the authors in this book. Consideration should also be given to providing incentives to health care providers to increase their attention to high-risk populations. Such incentives could, for example, provide higher compensation to providers of services to teenage mothers, based on best-practice guidelines. Overall, prioritizing policy initiatives should be influenced by quality-of-life outcomes and population health status rather than by short-term cost-effectiveness measures.

Third, improving the science base is necessary for improving adolescent health policy. In particular, identifying the mechanisms through which social determinants of health operate, and the theories that link these mechanisms, is crucial. Research is also needed to develop and test socio-cultural interventions that might affect adolescent health. Finally, assessments of the effect of policy (health and otherwise) on adolescent health are necessary. These health impact assessments, similar to environmental and gender impact assessments, consider a policy's likely intended and unintended consequences for health and use that information in the decision making process (Lurie 2002). The inclusion of the Institute for Human Development, Child and Youth Health in the Canadian Institutes of Health Research is an encouraging sign, although we would argue that the emphasis on adolescence is minimal at this point. This Institute could initially sponsor a report on adolescent health that identifies the key questions for research action. It could then sponsor a national funding competition on adolescent health that is widely based and stimulate innovation and confirmatory research on key adolescent health issues. For example, such a report and competition could assist in focusing a research agenda that would improve adolescent health by studying how social (family, peer, school, neighbourhood) environments affect adolescents' health. Similarly, CIHR and the Social Sciences and Humanities Research Council, which funds educational research, could sponsor a research theme on School Health.

Fourth, monitoring and reporting on key adolescent health indicators, as well as interventions, is necessary in order to see where we are going. The NLSCY and HBSC, in combination, allow examination of longitudinal cause-effect relationships and emerging cross-sectional prevalence indicators of adolescent health. These datasets provide useful information for monitoring program objectives, but there have been insufficient resources for their analysis. Joint efforts of Statistics Canada, Health Canada, CIHR, and the Canadian Institute for Health Information could provide such resources. Reports from both of these adolescent datasets should be routinely produced and widely disseminated. Linkages should be encouraged between the two national datasets as well as with other regional datasets (e.g., Better Beginnings Better Futures, Ontario) that deal with disadvantaged neighbourhoods. For all such reports, there needs to be a set of clear communication objectives and tools that increase their public educational value. Adolescent organizations, such as the Centre of Excellence for Youth Engagement, should be partners in this dissemination process so as to ensure that adolescent-friendly messages are produced.

Fifth, differentiation of policy approaches for adolescent health is advisable. Universal-type programs of social marketing and behaviour change for adolescents are designed to work at the population level. These may have the best chance of success with adolescents who, while keen to differentiate themselves in subcultures for the purposes of self-identity, are loath to subordinate other adolescents on the basis of their needs. At the same time, participatory targeted programs for adolescents who are estranged from family and school, living on the street in poverty, or raising their own children are crucial. Developing a sense of control and a meaningful role in such programs, rather than being "serviced" or receiving a handout, is vital for their acceptance and benefit to adolescents.

Finally, new linkages across sectors are necessary. Numerous federal, provincial, municipal, professional, and business sectors need to openly discuss the health of the next generation with adolescents themselves. An adolescent agenda in Canada would contribute to the visibility and viability of policy initiatives. A population health perspective is pointless if it does not focus on populations – women, children, ethnic minorities, Aboriginals, adolescents, and so on. Among these groups, adolescents have had little attention, in part because of their transitional character, independence seeking, and uneasy relationship with adults. The relationship of health ministries with other policy sectors should not be one-way (i.e., just recruiting the cooperation of others in developing new health policies). The formal health sector should also contribute its expertise when other bureaucracies are developing their own policies. Experts on adolescent issues must become more prominent in the policy field, as have experts in women's and children's issues. Standing committees on adolescence could take the coordinating lead in many jurisdictions. Alternatively, senior health officials could be assigned liaison responsibilities with each federal or provincial department and as staff on key parliamentary committees with responsibilities for policies likely to have a health effect on adolescents.

These initiatives, however, would need to demonstrate relatively rapid payoffs to be seen as adding value to the policy-making process.

CHALLENGES TO THESE RECOMMENDATIONS

There are a number of challenges to implementing this vision of adolescent health policy in Canada. Among these are: the relatively good health status of adolescents in Canadian society; a lack of government attention, in general, to social determinants of health in the long term; a lack of clarity and credibility in the health determinants message; continuing federal-provincial disagreements on health-care funding and appropriate levels of health care; and lack of an overall view on the relationship between health insurance, health care costs, and long-term health savings that may be achieved through addressing the social determinants of health.

As a preliminary comment, it is evident that adolescence is perceived as a generally healthy period of transition between childhood health problem risks and adult health problem certainties. Childhood health problems, for many reasons, have been given priority attention in the public's mind. Adult health problems, nonetheless, consume the majority of the health budget. Adolescence is largely seen as a period of relief from childhood health disasters, for which children are not held accountable. Adolescent health problems may be seen increasingly as the problems that young people create for themselves, primarily through risk-taking behaviours that lead to injury, such as smoking, sexual activity, and substance use, but also through the development of unhealthy, sedentary behaviour. From a health programmatic perspective, adolescence is largely a time for taking a break. Unfortunately, without life-course research, we do not know whether adolescence is a key critical period for prevention of future population-health problems.

Second, a lack of attention to long-term health patterns is evident. Investments in some initiatives (e.g., smoking cessation) to improve health, as noted previously, may reduce short-term costs of illness by avoiding complications, improving quality of life, and increasing life expectancy. Other initiatives intended to address physical inactivity, stress, and unhealthy eating habits may take decades to show a return. Some non-health initiatives (e.g., education) may take a generation to do so. Government attention has tended to focus on the short term, in part because of the divided public opinion on the role of any government in health promotion as opposed to health care.

A third dynamic is the lack of clarity in the health-determinants and health-policy messages over the past thirty-five years. From lifestyle approaches to health (1970s), to health promotion and community participation (1980s), to population health and public policy (1990s) the message has been constantly changing. Arguably, there have been studies (or, more accurately, policy prescriptions) to accompany each of these messages. There has been precious little research, however, to demonstrate the value of one approach over another (Lavis 2002). A related problem is the opportunism of politicians who espouse one message regarding health determinants, and who protect certain public health interests, while in one cabinet position (e.g., Health) and then change their views when in another position (e.g., Agriculture, Industry). The result is a lack of credibility in the entire message.

A fourth challenge is in the continuing jurisdictional disputes on health, in addition to those in other sectors, between federal and provincial policy-makers. While these disputes generally focus on health cost-sharing arrangements, they spill over into lack of cooperation on substantive health issues. The result is duplication of demonstration projects, especially in the area of health promotion, without the creation of clear links to other sectors (e.g., education, welfare, labour) that are responsible for coordinating actions.

Finally, there is a lack of public appreciation of the relationship between health insurance, health care costs, and health savings that are due to health promotion and prevention initiatives from multiple sectors. In Canada, a high value has been put on public health insurance (now made painless to the consumer as premiums are deducted at source and are often part of the employer's contributions). Health care costs are made invisible due to hospital/physician direct billing arrangements. The only place that consumers feel the "cost" of their health is through their general income tax rates and other sales taxes, and these are not differentiated to illustrate health costs. Consumers know that a significant portion of the federal and provincial budgets are used to pay for health care, but they do not know either the share of their tax dollar devoted to health or the cost to the economy in employer health insurance contributions. Coupled with these hidden figures, the severe lack of cost-effectiveness studies on health promotion interventions makes the possibility of health-promotion policy advances unlikely.

In conclusion, it is not a simple task to develop effective, coordinated, and localized adolescent health policy. The development of health policy that truly reflects the multiple and interacting determinants of health, and that truly reflects the various issues affecting different communities, populations, demographics, and age groups, is a costly and complex process. It is clear that, in order to meet the diversity of adolescents' needs across the country, and to ensure that adolescents' rights are fulfilled in all capacities, more research must be undertaken and more data compiled to identify what problems, needs, and human rights issues actually exist. Qualitative and survey research that listens to adolescents, and that respects self-reported health information, is of particular significance in fulfilling the principle of adolescent participation in policy development and decisions. This research must, however, be used in its full capacity – both to inform adolescent health policy and to evaluate its effectiveness.

Ideally, adolescent health and well-being in Canada can be improved through the successful coordination of evidence-based research, attention to rights, and policy.

REFERENCES

Health Canada. 1999. *Healthy Development of Children and Youth: The Role of the Determinants of Health*. Ottawa: Health Canada. http://www.phac-aspc.gc.ca/dca-dea/publications/healthy_dev_overview_e.html. Updated 2 September 2002. Retrieved 31 July 2007.

Lavis, J.N. 2002. Ideas at the margin or marginalized ideas? Non-medical determinants of health in Canada. *Health Affairs* 21 (2):107–12.

Lurie, N. 2002. What the federal government can do about the non-medical determinants of health. *Health Affairs* 21(2):94–106.

Index